'In a time that is nothing less than ongoing "radical reorientation," Spiritual Direction and the Other challenges us to turn toward our differences to find new ground for cultivating meaning and hope. Pressing beyond the often hyper-individualized medical or spiritual constructs of both psychology and spirituality, Daniels, Capretto, and Vogel gather a chorus of expert voices to assist in this inherently communal work. The volume bridges secular and faith-based research and practice, making the "other side" legible across professional and religious boundaries. It offers ambitious yet accessible chapters on a wide range of topics, pushing the field of spiritual direction in particular to face what it must do to meet this moment. This volume will be essential for pastoral formation classrooms, practitioners across the helping professions, interreligious leaders, and those of us who, in some way, care for people in all their complexity – ours and others – and desire to do so from an orientation of psychological as well as spiritual best practices.'

Stephanie C. Edwards, *MSW, PhD, Executive Director, Boston Theological Interreligious Consortium and Adjunct Faculty, Boston College*

'Drawing on the Desert Fathers and Mothers of the early Christian tradition, Franciscan and Ignatian spiritualities, as well as on Buddhist discourse, Afro-Caribbean humanism, personal and classroom experiences of the authors, the insights of philosophy, psychology, counselling and psychotherapy, this unique collection of essays takes a creatively broad view of the processes of discernment at the heart of the practice of spiritual direction. It brings critical academic rigour and, at the same time, an awareness of the "limits of worldly knowledge" and an apophatic appreciation of the encounter with the other in "holy darkness". Critical, spiritual and reflective; highly recommended!'

Christopher Cook, BSc, MB, BS, MD, MA, PhD, FRCPsych, *Emeritus Professor in the Department of Theology and Religion, Durham University and Reverend Professor in the Institute for Medical Humanities, Durham University*

Spiritual Direction and the Other

Spiritual Direction and the Other offers the first interdisciplinary exploration of how ancient traditions of spiritual accompaniment can restore openness to mystery and cultural sensitivity in our psychotherapeutic helping professions.

As therapeutic culture has grown to dominate the landscape of helping professions in recent decades, humanistic caregivers have increasingly struggled to identify methods and traditions that remain open to the Other. Though often neglected by mainstream psychology, spiritual direction not only provides an alternative mode of accompanying others in a world of growing instability, but also draws from an intellectual history that predates the earliest Western medical and psychological theories by centuries. This edited collection is the first to explore the history of spiritual direction as a resource for both accompanying others with cultural sensitivity and resisting the hegemony of reductionism in psychotherapy. Its authors invite readers into sacred, and sometimes unsettling, conversations about how we accompany others through crises of meaning-making, trauma, and pluralistic longing. Whether engaging Desert Fathers and Mothers, Spanish mystics, Afro-Caribbean humanism, Buddhist pedagogy, contemporary psychoanalysis, or Italian literary arts, its contributors offer distinct encounters with what it means to listen for the sacred in the strange, the suffering, and the soul.

Bringing together interdisciplinary contributors from clinical psychology, theology, philosophy, chaplaincy, and history, this volume provides not only a rich analysis of the identity of spiritual direction in the 21st century, but models of how spiritual direction can inform caregiving, advocacy and education in countless contexts.

Aaron B. Daniels is Teaching Professor in the Psychology Department at Northeastern University, USA. He is the editor of *A Phenomenology of the Alien: Encounters with the Weird and Inscrutable Other* (2025) and *Dante and the Other: A Phenomenology of Love* (2021).

Peter Capretto is Associate Professor of Psychology, Culture, and Religion at Phillips Theological Seminary, USA. His writings on the philosophy and psychology of religion have appeared in over a dozen scholarly journals and books.

Gracie Vogel graduated from Northeastern University with a B.S. in Health Science and Psychology.

Psychology and the Other

Series editor: David M. Goodman
Associate editors: Matthew Clemente, Brian W. Becker, Donna M. Orange and Eric R. Severson

The *Psychology and the Other* book series highlights creative work at the intersections between psychology and the vast array of disciplines relevant to the human psyche. The interdisciplinary focus of this series brings psychology into conversation with continental philosophy, psychoanalysis, religious studies, anthropology, sociology, and social/critical theory. The cross-fertilization of theory and practice, encompassing such a range of perspectives, encourages the exploration of alternative paradigms and newly articulated vocabularies that speak to human identity, freedom, and suffering. Thus, we are encouraged to reimagine our encounters with difference, our notions of the "other," and what constitutes therapeutic modalities.

The study and practices of mental health practitioners, psychoanalysts, and scholars in the humanities will be sharpened, enhanced, and illuminated by these vibrant conversations, representing pluralistic methods of inquiry, including those typically identified as psychoanalytic, humanistic, qualitative, phenomenological, or existential.

Recent titles in the series include:

Spiritual Direction and the Other
Interdisciplinary Explorations of Accompaniment
Aaron B. Daniels, Peter Capretto and Gracie Vogel

Winnicott's Psychoanalysis of Being
Emotional Development as Phenomenology-Based Psychology
Leopoldo Fulgencio

Fanon and Lacan
Decolonial Psychoanalysis
Derek Hook & Sinan Richards

For a full list of titles in the series, please visit the Routledge website at: https://www.routledge.com/Psychology-and-the-Other/book-series/PSYOTH

Spiritual Direction and the Other

Interdisciplinary Explorations of Accompaniment

Edited by
Aaron B. Daniels, Peter Capretto and
Gracie Vogel

Routledge
Taylor & Francis Group
LONDON AND NEW YORK

Designed cover image: Getty Images

First published 2027
by Routledge
4 Park Square, Milton Park, Abingdon, Oxon OX14 4RN

and by Routledge
605 Third Avenue, New York, NY 10158

Routledge is an imprint of the Taylor & Francis Group, an informa business

British Library Cataloguing-in-Publication Data
A catalogue record for this book is available from the British Library

Library of Congress Cataloging-in-Publication Data
A catalog record has been requested for this book

ISBN: 978-1-041-24634-3 (hbk)
ISBN: 978-1-041-24633-6 (pbk)
ISBN: 978-1-003-74285-2 (ebk)

DOI: 10.4324/9781003742852

Typeset in Times New Roman
by Taylor & Francis Books

Contents

Tables

Contributors

Corné J. Bekker serves as professor and the Dean of the School of Divinity at Regent University in Virginia Beach, Virginia. In addition to these roles, he is the Director of the ThM and PhD programs in Renewal Theology at Regent University.

Gordon Bermant is Senior Research Associate with the American Buddhist Study Center. Working from Philadelphia, his primary role is to further public understanding of Shin Buddhism (Nishi) in the United States. He attempts to avoid taking himself too seriously.

Peter Capretto, PhD, is Associate Professor of Psychology, Culture, and Religion at Phillips Theological Seminary. He is author of *Beyond the Empathy Trap: Cultivating Freedom and Solidarity* in an Ethic of Care (2026) and co-editor of *Trauma and Transcendence: Suffering and the Limits of Theory* (2018).

Vanessa Cha graduated *summa cum laude* with a BSc in Psychology and a minor in Public Health from Northeastern University. Her work at the Harvard Meditation Research Program explored risk factors for emergent phenomena. She currently resides in Vancouver, guiding meditations at a women's shelter while exploring graduate school options.

The **Rev. Pamela Cooper-White**, PhD, is the Christiane Brooks Johnson Professor Emerita of Psychology and Religion at Union Theological Seminary, and author of ten books including *Shared Wisdom: Use of the Self in Pastoral Care and Counseling*, now in its second edition. She is an ordained Episcopal priest, psychoanalytic psychotherapist, and spiritual director.

Anthony Cruz Pantojas, a PhD candidate in Cultural Studies (Universidad Ana G. Méndez, Puerto Rico), is a scholar-practitioner and Board-Certified Chaplain serving as Associate University Chaplain at Tufts University. An ordained Animal Chaplain and certified Spiritual Director, Cruz Pantojas cultivates a creolizing approach to existential care grounded in Afro-Caribbean theory.

Aaron B. Daniels, PhD is Teaching Professor, Mindfulness Fellow, and leader of the Psychological Humanities Research Group at Northeastern

University in Boston, Massachusetts. He is the editor of *A Phenomenology of the Alien: Encounters with the Weird and Inscrutable Other* (2025) and *Dante and the Other: A Phenomenology of Love* (2021).

Alden Flanders is a priest of the Episcopal Church and a spiritual director at Bethany House of Prayer in Arlington, Massachusetts. His undergraduate work was done at Hobart College. He holds graduate degrees in theater, divinity, and education, and has worked as a parish priest and a boarding school teacher.

Katherine E. Kirby, PhD, is a Professor of Philosophy and Equity Studies at Saint Michael's College, Vermont. She serves as Director of the Equity Studies Program and Director of the Junior Seminar Program. Dr. Kirby specializes in theoretical and applied ethics, community-engaged learning, and theories of oppression, resistance, and liberation.

Gracie Vogel graduated *summa cum laude* from Northeastern University with a B.S. in Health Science and Psychology and a minor in Journalism. She has worked in research at Dana-Farber Cancer Institute and Brigham and Women's Hospital. She lives in Boston and is hoping to pursue a career in public health.

Jonathan L. Zecher is an Associate Professor of Early and Byzantine Christian Studies at the Australian Catholic University. He studies primarily Greek monastic literature, ancient medicine, and the history of emotions. In 2022 he published *Spiritual Direction as a Medical Art in Early Christian Monasticism*.

Acknowledgements

This volume emerged from a "Spiritual Direction Salon" at the 2023 Psychology and the Other Conference held at Boston College. We are deeply grateful to David Goodman and the Center for Psychological Humanities and Ethics for believing in the idea that bringing together spiritual directors and thinkers from a range of religions, perspectives, and practices was a worthy undertaking.

The group that would become Psychological Humanities at Northeastern University was essential in running that conference and making the Spiritual Direction Salon such a rich success. Many thanks to the 16 students who volunteered.

The polyphony of that original gathering rings throughout this collection and we are deeply thankful to the contributors who have offered their chapters.

One does not come to devote time and effort to the practice and study of spiritual direction without having become marvelously entangled in the spiritual journeys of friends, families, colleagues, and mentors. To all of them, we offer a deep bow of thanks.

Finally, to those "friends of the heart," those "soul's friends" who have been our closest companions on this journey, we dedicate this volume.

Aaron B. Daniels
(Northeastern University, Boston, Massachusetts)
Peter Capretto
(Phillips Theological Seminary, Tulsa, Oklahoma)
Gracie Vogel
(Northeastern University, Boston, Massachusetts)

Chapter 1

Introduction

"Exploring the Other in Spiritual Direction"

Aaron B. Daniels, Peter Capretto and Gracie Vogel

When compared to the history and evolution of psychotherapy, spiritual direction reveals itself to be a peculiar and perhaps even dangerous supplement. Within the context of an ever-expanding disciplinary landscape where novel helping modalities constantly vie for unique territory to call their own, spiritual direction occupies an odd temporal space, presenting as both a new-age alternative to Western psychotherapies and yet historically predating them by a healthy measure. Spiritual direction is an old tradition that was reflecting on how to accompany others through their most vexing life challenges for millennia before Freud hit the scene. And while spiritual direction's history has undergone its own permutations, it has not been contested, defended, and revolutionized with the same frequency as other forms of dyadic accompaniment. This discordant juxtaposition raises a curious puzzle for 21st-century helping professionals and theorists: either spiritual direction's long tradition has already taken an inventory of the dialectical tension that psychotherapy is still working through, or spiritual direction is overdue for subversion.

The intrigue regarding spiritual direction's history and future would remain purely theoretical if not for the time of crisis its practitioners find themselves in today. It is not simply that helping professions are now wrestling with the encroachment of political and systemic violences into the often individualistically constructed context of a therapeutic exchange; progressive and socially mindful psychotherapists have observed for decades that one cannot bracket the influences of late capitalism from the testimony of the couch. Rather, it is sober recognition that the classical psychoanalytic ambition to transform neurotic misery into everyday unhappiness may all but ensure societal and ecological demise. Environmentalists inform us of the gravity of global climate change. Psychiatric epidemiologists sound the alarm of vast swathes of societies caught between mounting mental health struggles and inadequate or non-existent resources, contributing to the changing face of ever-looming addiction struggles. Social activists take to the streets to tell us of the brutal structural inequalities of our societies. War rages across the globe and shell-shocked refugees live in abject, interstitial anxiety. That we live in an age of crisis is one of the few things competing politicians can agree on.

DOI: 10.4324/9781003742852-1

Yet as novel and genuinely dangerous as these existential threats may be, one humbling insight of the long history of spiritual direction is that it takes a special form of myopia to insist that the crisis of one's present moment is unique. The challenge is to contextualize without trivialization: these crises are indeed world threatening and draw upon emerging technologies for destruction never seen before; and others have gone before you with structurally similar prospects of annihilation. Apocalyptic literature within Abrahamic traditions stretches back to at least the 6th century BCE and continued for a millennium or more. Although these dramatic texts typically seem to be predictions of a cataclysmic future, they are also most often figurative descriptions of the tumultuous world of the writers' present times. Regardless of their original intent, these visions of the end of the world continue to resonate for some readers who see in them reflections of the world-on-fire around them today. This is similar to the way psalms of mourning and lamentation speak to what is too-often the world of the marginalized and oppressed.

This age of crisis brings with it a grinding toll on its denizens. Today, the word trauma has broadened well beyond its psychiatric definition which necessitates threat of death, severe injury, or violation. The language of stress, suffering, sorrow, moral injury, or woundedness just doesn't seem to carry the necessary weight nor clinical authority. So, we speak of educational, relationship, familial, religious, cultural, environmental, and emotional trauma, to name a few. We speak also of how we inherit—culturally and epigenetically—intergenerational trauma from events of which we may never have heard.

In the face of all these crises, responses often fall into two broad camps: what we're doing is helping, but we need to do more; or we're looking at the problem all wrong. The first perspective asserts that we have the answers readily available to us now and the real problem is that we have not adequately doubled down on them. Thus, to put it more pointedly: we will be able to cap-and-trade our way out of global climate change. We just need enough mental health professionals to address our suffering. We can create enough legislation to change racist, sexist, hetero- and cis-normative cultures. We just need to elect the right person to turn the corner on these many crises. Economic sanctions, strategic arms deals, and just the right application of the ravages of war finally will rid the world of injustice and bring peace. And the suppression of hot wars brings the required breathing room to truly achieve peace and the ability to address these other struggles.

Both the "we need to do more" and the "we need to do differently" perspectives deny that the state of the world and its further decay are inevitable. But the call to see and be differently rejects the belief that the dominant approaches to addressing these challenges would work if we just pushed a little harder. Instead, believing that current efforts are not appropriate to these crises, we are left to ask: what do we believe we need to do to make the sort of fundamental changes to alter the course of history?

In Greek, "apocalypse" [ἀποκάλυψις] means something like "unveiling." One could think of this as a sort of showing what was always, already there. Can one's crises be an invitation, a demand to look again, to look differently, to look more deeply? In the discernment of spiritual direction, all of this can happen only by learning to overtly orient ourselves toward that which most matters to us. In doing so, one assesses how one takes that up, and one judges how to measure up to that. One changes how one sees. In doing so, one can change where one's gaze rests. What truly matters most to me now that I see differently?

Spiritual Direction as Discerning Apocalypse

Darkness is a fundamental metaphor of spiritual direction. Saint John of the Cross enshrines it in his *Dark Night of the Soul*—originally a poem written between 1577 and 1579, followed by his commentary created 1584–1586. Poets, theologians, and spiritual directors—not mutually exclusive categories—make frequent use of this dark night metaphor, usually intending it as a synonym for crisis—something like a test of faith. However, this is not the only available interpretation. John is, after all, a poet and mystic with apophatic leanings. That is, he deeply questions whether we can make positive rational statements about the nature of God and even the nature of reality. Thus, it is also possible to take this dark night as a star-filled place of wonder. This can be similar to the sacrament of silence many Quakers observe. This holy darkness can be a statement on how little we actually can know—and how little value our knowledge truly offers unto itself. To put philosophical jargon onto it: John is offering us a statement about the real limitations of our epistemologies. How we know—or think we know—is far less extensive than we typically seem capable of acknowledging. Only in embracing the profound limits of our knowledge may we open up to the greater reality in which we are truly living every moment of our lives.

Thus, with the limits of our worldly knowledge and the potential for a holy darkness in mind, we can revisit our Age of Crisis. Might not the sort of sweeping changes necessary to alter the course of history demand individuals take up their lives in radically different ways? We frequently speak of changing our minds—whether the actual shifts are common or not. Most people would report that they do change their minds when given adequate evidence. Yet, when it comes to hearts and souls, we more often speak of listening to our hearts or finding soulmates, baring our souls, or old souls. These heart and soul idioms decidedly drift more poetic. Thus, what sort of evidence could we rely upon even to know our hearts, mind our hearts, or care for our souls?

A core element of spiritual direction is discernment. In discernment, we learn to listen more deeply—to ourselves, to others, and, within the Judeo-Christian tradition, to the "still small voice" (*1 Kings* 19:12, KJV). We learn to listen deeply in spiritual direction, because our companion, the director, listens so deeply to us. Over time, we come to know that we may well have spent much of our lives ignoring, dismissing, or expressing overt hostility to a wide range of evidence our lives have offered us. Pleasure and discomfort, pain and longing, loneliness and being overwhelmed, hope and despair, intuitions and fear—we discover these sources of evidence through a deep subjectivity. In spiritual direction we cultivate types of awareness: in prayer, meditation, and other contemplative practices; through reading and writing poetry; through the stories we tell and the stories that move us; through conversations that make us laugh, make us mad, bring us to tears; through dreams and fantasies; through the sublime in art and in our broken world. And we practice all these skills with someone who is striving to do the same with us and themselves.

Situating this Volume within the Literature of Spiritual Direction

Because of the oft-repeated story that spiritual direction has its origins in the early Christian Desert Fathers and Mothers in the 3rd to 5th centuries CE, Merton's *The Wisdom of the Desert: Sayings of the Desert Fathers of the Fourth Century* (1960) is a frequently assigned reading in spiritual direction training. Within this current volume, Jonathan Zecher magisterially takes up this provenance and, by way of John Cassian's (c. 360–435 CE) descriptions of the Desert Fathers, provides a pre-Christian foundation for spiritual direction in ancient Greek medicine and philosophy. In their responses, Peter Capretto and Aaron B. Daniels each take the perspectives Zecher raises and extend them into questions of soulfulness and mortality.

Growing from the tone of the Desert Fathers and Mothers, mystical themes are often implicit in spiritual direction texts. An abiding sub-stream in curricula, overt mysticism often reaches back to medieval Christian works. This can be seen in the frequency with which *The Cloud of Unknowing and the Book of Privy Counseling* from the 14th century (e.g., Johnston's 1973 translation of the anonymous work) appears as assigned or supplemental reading—or the use of comprehensive surveys and commentaries on mysticism such as Evelyn Underhill's (1875–1941) three volumes from 1911, 1914, and 1920 (Underhill, 2017).

Mystical themes dominate the core of the historical portion of reading lists rooted in the works of the Christian religious figures from the Middle Ages into the Enlightenment who served as spiritual directors. These include Julian of Norwich's (1343–1416) *Revelations of Divine Love* (Julian of Norwich, 2015), Teresa of Ávila's (1515–1582) *The Interior Castle* (Teresa of Ávila, 2020), the aforementioned Saint John of the Cross's (1542–1591) *Dark Night of the Soul* (John of the Cross, 1964), and, of course, one cannot avoid Ignatius of Loyola's (1491–1556) *Spiritual Exercises* (Ignatius of Loyola, 1999 [1522–1524]). This last Jesuit approach is an entire class of spiritual direction unto itself with commentaries and personal accounts abounding since the work's publication (e.g., Nadal, 2005 [1593]; Harbaugh, 1997; O'Brien, 2011; Salai, 2020). Arguably, Barry and Connolly's (2009) *The Practice of Spiritual Direction* extends the Jesuit perspective into a fuller vision of spiritual direction beyond the formal structure of Ignatius's *Exercises.* Claiming an older origin, but not an avowed spiritual director, Dante Alighieri (1260–1321) often receives passing mention in texts—as he does in Daniels's response to Zecher in this volume; nevertheless, Paul Pearson's three volumes (Pearson, 2019, 2020, 2022) mapping spiritual direction onto Dante's *Commedia* stand alone. In this current book, Corné Bekker stretches deeper into the Middle Ages and provides a profound textual analysis of Clare of Assisi's (1194–1253) spiritual direction as found in her correspondences with a directee.

With chapters by Gordon Bermant, Katherine Kirby, and Vanessa Cha, this volume extends into Buddhist discourse in a more pronounced way than one typically sees in books explicitly about "spiritual direction." This failure to integrate Buddhist perspectives is likely because of the term's deep history in Christianity, and its development within medieval Western Christian practice. As professional organizations—such as Spiritual Directors International, founded in 1990—have grown and expanded into interfaith discourse, many Buddhist clergy and leaders have noted close parallels between Christian practice and Buddhist mindfulness and meditation mentoring. Of course, in the West, the literature of mindfulness and meditation is a massive corpus from over the last 60 years. Yet the books are often guides for individual practices and their definitions and methodologies vary widely.

Bermant, Kirby, and Cha all integrate their own stories and transformations into their accounts. Bermant invites readers to consider how a deeper examination of Christian doctrine and practice can bring one to the same frontiers to which the Buddhist journeys. Kirby examines that widely-practiced but scarcely acknowledged form of group spiritual direction: college humanities courses—in this case, a course on meditation and social justice. Kirby also provides a strong list of references to support these sorts of classroom experiences. Cha weaves her own story with a thorough examination of ongoing research into the unusual phenomena that can emerge in meditation, and how supportive mentoring, such as spiritual direction, can help contain and guide these experiences.

This current volume is not exhaustive in its perspectives. Nonetheless, collected volumes are relatively rare in the literature of spiritual direction. Although individual authors offer ample and poetic takes on the practice of spiritual direction—far exceeding the capacity of any literature review to encapsulate—collected volumes allow themes to deepen through contrasting perspectives and can invite further scholarship. Moon and Benner (2004) gather seven essays from Christian clergy on sometimes radically different visions of spiritual direction. The editors follow this inventory with six authors considering the boundaries and overlap between direction, psychotherapy, and pastoral counseling. In a more recent collection, Adesanya (2019) draws together 12 spiritual directors of color, mostly women, to offer many perspectives on spiritual direction that—in the 15 years since Moon and Beener (2004)—pitch to a distinctly broader sense of the art.

Like Adesanya (2019), Taylor-Stinson (2017) collects essays from a range of voices, including a chapter by Adesanya, to more specifically explore the integral relationship between contemplation and social justice. Peacock (2020) continues weaving that tapestry by providing profiles of ten African American spiritual leaders, followed by exercises to aid the reader in engaging with the challenges and wisdom these perspectives raise. These works find that advocacy demands spiritual care of oneself—and that spiritual care for oneself calls one to advocacy. Thus, Howard Thurman (1899–1981) looms large in all these works, in particular his 1949 masterpiece *Jesus and the Disinherited* (Thurman, 1949). In our current volume, Anthony Cruz Pantojas challenges us to think and feel far more deeply into the many forms of difference—around constructions of race, culture, neurodiversity, gender, and sexual orientation, to name just a few—that invite us to grow and transform in our relationship to the other and the Other.

A trend found throughout many if not most texts addressing spiritual direction is the struggle with definition that we too take up above. Where does it sit in relationship with psychotherapy, pastoral counseling, life coaching, and more? In many ways, psychiatrist Gerald May (1940–2005) inaugurates this conversation in his oft-assigned text *Care of Mind/Care of Spirit* (May, 1982). He then weaves these themes throughout many of his subsequent works including *Addiction and Grace* (May, 1988) and *The Dark Night of the Soul* (May, 2004). In 1973, May joined the group created by Tilden Edwards that would become the Shalem Institute for Spiritual Formation in Bethesda, Maryland. Shalem has exercised a strong influence over the shape of spiritual direction and the discourse around it in the U.S. for many decades.

Thus, it is a true gift that Pamela Cooper-White offers a chapter in this collection in which she incisively returns to fundamental questions about the relationship at the heart of spiritual direction. Cooper-White creates a dialogue between psychoanalytic thought and spiritual direction to help deconstruct assumptions that may have outlived their utility. Also drawing on psychoanalytic insights as well as literary and philological perspectives, Alden Flanders asks directors to see the space of encounter as an invitation to realize the fundamental metaphors we each live. These accounts from two individuals who think deeply about the practice itself give ample room for the tension and struggles with which directors and directees alike must sit. As such, although drawing on different sources, the depth and compassion of their writings place Cooper-White and Flanders as part of the tradition that finds heart-breaking voice in the works of Henri Nouwen (1932–1996) (e.g., Nouwen, 1992) and sings in the writings of John O'Donahue (1956–2008) (e.g., O'Donahue, 1997).

Conclusion

Our hopes are that this volume provides not only a rich historical and theoretical tapestry for advanced researchers in the humanities and health professions around spiritual direction, but also a wealth of practical and clinically oriented resources for those participating in the long tradition of accompanying others in spiritual direction. Given the growing apocalypses that continue to impact the health, wellness, and security of so many persons as we venture further into the 21st century, we hope that this collection also may provide a glimpse or unveiling of a deeper way of seeing our lives and the lives of the other.

References

Anonymous (1973). *The cloud of unknowing and the book of privy counseling* (W. Johnston, Trans.). Image Classics. (Original work published c. late 14th century.)

Adesanya, I. P. (Ed.) (2019). *Kaleidoscope: Broadening the palette in the art of Spiritual Direction.* Church Publishing Incorporated.

Barry, W. A., and Connolly, W. J. (2009). *The practice of spiritual direction* (revised and updated). HarperCollins.

Harbaugh, J. (1997). *A 12-step approach to the Spiritual Exercises of St. Ignatius.* Sheed and Ward.

Ignatius of Loyola. (1999). *The Spiritual Exercises of St. Ignatius: or Manresa.* TAN Books. (Original work published 1522–1524.)

John of the Cross. (1964). *The complete works of St. John of the Cross* (K. Kavanaugh & O. Rodriguez, Trans.). Thomas Nelson and Sons.

Julian of Norwich. (2015). *Revelations of divine love* (B. Windeatt, Trans.). Oxford World Classics. (Original work written between 14th to 15th centuries.)

May, G. G. (1982). *Care of mind/Care of spirit: A psychiatrist explores spiritual direction.* Harper and Row.

May, G. G. (1988) *Addiction and grace: Love and spirituality in the healing of addictions.* Harper and Row.

May, G. G. (2004). *Dark night of the soul: A psychiatrist explores the connections between darkness and spiritual growth.* Harper and Row.

Merton, T. (1960). *The wisdom of the desert: Sayings of the Desert Fathers of the fourth century.* New Directions Books.

Moon, G. W. and Benner, D. G. (Eds.) (2004). *Spiritual direction and the care of souls: A guide to Christian approaches and practices.* IVP Academic.

Nadal, J. (2005). *Illustrated Spiritual Exercises.* University of Scranton Press. (Original work published 1593.)

Nouwen, H. J. M. (1992). *The return of the prodigal son.* Doubleday.

O'Brien, K. (2011). *The Ignatian adventure: Experiencing the Spiritual Exercises of St. Ignatius in daily life.* Loyola Press.

O'Donohue, J. (1997). *Anam cara: A book of Celtic wisdom.* Cliff Street Books.

Peacock, B. L. (2020). *Soul care in African American practice.* IVP Formatio.

Pearson, P. (2019). *Spiritual direction from Dante: Avoiding the Inferno (Volume 1).* TAN Books.

Pearson, P. (2020). *Spiritual direction from Dante: Ascending Mount Purgatory (Volume 2)*. TAN Books.
Pearson, P. (2022). *Spiritual direction from Dante: Yearning for Paradise (Volume 3)*. TAN Books.
Salai, S. M. (2020). *The Spiritual Exercises of St. Ignatius of Loyola: With points for personal prayer from Jesuit spiritual masters*. TAN Books.
Taylor-Stinson, T. (Ed.). (2017). *Ain't gonna let nobody turn me around: Stories of contemplation and justice*. Church Publishing.
Teresa of Ávila. (2020). *The interior castle* (Second, study edition) (K. Kavanaugh and O. Rodriguez, Trans.). ICS Publications.
Thurman, H. (1949). *Jesus and the disinherited*. Abingdon Press.
Underhill, E. (2017). *Evelyn Underhill's three books on mysticism*. Neo Books. (Original works published 1911, 1914, and 1920.)

Chapter 2

Organizing Emotions and Challenging Values in Spiritual Direction

A Few Thoughts from the Christian Desert

Jonathan L. Zecher

John Cassian (c. 360–435 CE), in the last of his *Conferences*, recalls a moment during his youthful sojourn in Egypt among the great and good of the Desert Fathers. He says that he and his friend Germanus "carried in an anxious confession to Abba Abraham the assault of our daily thoughts, which urged us, with boiling emotions in our soul, to return to our own country and visit our parents" (24.1.2).[1] In response, Abba Abraham first elicits the reasons for these homesick thoughts, and then, pulling no punches, tells the younger monks that "the infirmity of your thoughts reveals the superficiality of your renunciation," while "the wandering of your desires bears witness to the slackness of your heart" (24.2.1). Abraham urges them to recover the fervor and desire that first led them to the desert, which should draw them to God through the rigors of monastic life. But he also spends some time explaining the origins of their various thoughts and emotions. He explains that "the source and beginning of all vices is the same, but it branches into different designations of the passions and corruptions according to the characteristics of that part in the soul that was damaged" (24.15.1). Abraham goes on to explore the various passions that Germanus and Cassian face and offers remedies appropriate to each.

In this story, Cassian, imagining himself again as a young monk talking with his Abba, shows us spiritual direction at work in the Egyptian desert—a hierarchical, unabashedly asymmetrical relationship of power and submission, discipline and obedience, of which the pivot is confession. At the same time, as I argue at length in *Spiritual Direction as a Medical Art in Early Christian Monasticism* (Zecher, 2022), this relationship is explicitly and relentlessly characterized as healing, as medicine, as diagnosis, and as therapy. Cassian's picture of spiritual direction presumes hierarchies, an all-encompassing form of life, and crosses boundaries into therapeutics and medicine. In each of these ways, Cassian's—and much of early monastic literature's—picture of spiritual direction stands apart from the companionable, frequently temporary, and deliberately non-medical modes of contemporary spiritual direction. Thus, time with Cassian, whom I have volunteered to stand in for much of the early Christian monastic tradition, challenges assumptions around the purpose, the mode, and the scope of spiritual direction.

DOI: 10.4324/9781003742852-2

In short, monks are good to think with. They help us question the assumptions underlying contemporary approaches to spiritual direction, consider its relations to psychotherapy and analysis, and begin making sense of a plurality of religious and secular forms of life implicated in modes of direction.

A Brief Outline

To tease out these challenges and possibilities raised by Cassian and other Desert Christians, I focus on the central role played by emotions—or "passions"—in enabling or obstructing the form of life that direction aims at. For Cassian, as we shall see, emotions mediate between the whirl of daily thoughts and the last dispositions which stand in need of transformation and growth if the monk is to draw near to God and others. This focus helps set Cassian in conversation with contemporary theories of cognition, sociality, and even biomedicine, which feature emotions as constitutive elements of embodied human existence. While the forms of life may differ, the materials of those lives are shared.

Following this line, I'll begin with some explanation of *why* I think we should think with monks like Cassian, by showing that ancient thinking on passions has much to say to contemporary ideas of emotion. It further directs us to embodiment and enculturation as key determinants of emotional experience. I will then turn to lists as means of articulating emotional repertoires and enforcing emotional regimes. In particular, ancient Stoic lists mediated between psychological causality and everyday experience, and early Christians drew on these as they developed their own emotional regimes. Coming then to Cassian and the early Christian desert, I will show how he develops lists from Evagrios of Pontus (c. 345–399 CE) to articulate a wide range of emotions and emotional dysfunction, to access underlying *affectus* [dispositions], and to transform these through confession and penance. I will show that dispositions, however, are themselves rooted in values and attachments, the configuration of which define the self. The end of emotional transformation is a more total self-transformation. The monastic self that emerges in Cassian's program is one suited by emotional habits both for the monastic community and the Kingdom of Heaven. I'll close by drawing out challenges implicit in the aims, mode, and regime of Cassian's—and other monastic—spiritual direction, to invite further reflection on the broader issues of plurality and value operative in modern spiritual direction.

Initial Soundings: Emotions Now and Passions Then

This chapter begins from the assumption that, despite differences of language, ancient "passions" refer to much the same phenomena as modern "emotions." A nice summary of the reasons behind this statement can be found in Champion et al.'s (2019) "But were they talking about the emotions? Affectus, affectio and the history of emotions." Rather than picking a definition of emotion from the many currently on offer, and still less trying to write my own, I want only to highlight two points of contact between several theories of emotion today and definitions from antiquity, both of which are salient to Cassian's project in spiritual direction.

First, contemporary theories of emotion in philosophy and psychology are componential. In being so, they track ancient ones in having an evaluative component: whether perceptual (Tappolet, 2016) or judgemental (Solomon, 1976; Nussbaum, 2001); an action-readiness component (Frijda, 1986; 2006); as well as an affective or feeling one.[2] Thus, for example, when the ancients defined a "passion" like anger as both "desire for revenge" (see Pseudo-Andronicus, 1884, "On the Passions," 1.4, p. 17; and Laertius, 1925, p. 218, 7.113) and "the boiling of blood around the heart,"[3] they too were thinking in components. Moreover, these components set emotions within a social and embodied space, creating narratives in which people find themselves not only feeling, but perceiving, judging, and ultimately, acting in certain ways.

Second, emotions now as then are motivational, and morally evaluated. Emotions make us want to act in certain ways because we want certain outcomes (Frijda, 2016; or for a view of motivation that does not require cognitivist theory, see Scarantino, 2014). This is essential. In turn, we praise or blame people for their emotional self-control or lack thereof, we evaluate the appropriateness of a given emotion in a given situation, and so on. The sometimes-negative picture of emotion that is associated with ancient philosophies, especially Stoic and Christian, results from their moral evaluation of certain kinds of emotion. We'll see that Cassian is far from negative about emotion as such, but he does strongly condemn certain kinds of emotional styles and dispositions.

At the same time, ancient ideas of emotion trouble contemporary theories in several ways. These points of difference or pushback are at least as important, I think, for why we should take time to think with early monks. Ancient "passions" include emotions—anger, sadness, jealousy, joy, delight, hope, and so on—but also include things like hunger, exhaustion, growth, and ageing. Emotions were understood as species of embodied, contingent, human experience, in that regard both natural and challenging. These "natural passions" could easily shade into morally reprehensible ones, as hunger becomes gluttony, thirst becomes drunkenness, exhaustion becomes laziness, and so on. There was, therefore, a constant moral concern around autonomy within the constraints of inbuilt passivity. This concern motivates much monastic thinking on passions, in part because it allows Cassian and others to foreground emotions as emblematic of broader human experience, and as mediating all sorts of deeper dispositions and values into action and thought. Cassian can then use the transformation of emotional dispositions as a way of catalysing a whole form of life. Monastic emotional practices are, really, about claiming agency within embodied constraints. Cassian (see *Conferences*, 4.11.1–4.15.2) likes to frame this as the will vacillating between the desires of flesh and those of the spirit—and he is clear that, while it may seem best to choose only things of the spirit, one must care for the body, cherish it even. And so the constraints of embodiment serve as the boundary markers for the monastic struggle.

At the same time, emotions are culturally conditioned, if not culturally produced. In Batja Mesquita's (2022) phrasing, modern theories of emotion have often treated them as "MINE" or "Mental, INside, and Essentialist," which suggests that emotions are hardwired and individual for the very reason they are universal. Mesquita, along with other more recent theorists in neuroscience and social psychology, pushes us instead to think that emotions are "OURS": "OUtside, Relational, and Situated." In this model, emotions are shared to the same degree and for the same reason that they are culturally contingent. Historians of emotion have long recognized this and have shown moreover that emotional styles are enforced and disciplined within communities, part of the shared symbolic language of a given culture, becoming what William Reddy (2001) called "emotional regimes" in which individuals are formed and within which they must participate. These regimes are, inevitably, classed, gendered, and conditioned by the unspoken prejudices and symbolic systems of the culture within which they are formed. Those unspoken prejudices are easier for the historian to recover than for the person on the ground to recognize. So too as we look to Cassian, we will see a preference for a certain kind of masculinity and a hierarchical sociality that may seem quite foreign—and yet, if those are his assumptions, we may then ask, what are ours?

Emotions are, then, embodied and en-cultured, located within a broader array of vulnerabilities and passivities contingent on embodied experience. Just so, social and cultural cues both organize and enforce social norms in emotion. Language of emotion is integral to all of this, as naming emotions contributes both to articulating, and to regulating them (Scheer, 2012). This brings us back to spiritual direction: emotional experience is at the heart of human life, crossing supposed boundaries between cognitive, affective, and practical operations. That experience is likewise conditioned, evaluated, and disciplined by the community of relationships within which the individual is suspended. The attempt, displayed in monastic literature and memory, to transform emotion is, I would suggest, an attempt to refashion the human being ready for a new and, indeed, transcendent form of life. So, how was this done?

Lists and Their Uses

Neuroscientists and philosophers alike are realizing more and more the role played by emotion language in emotional experience. Some, like Lisa Feldman Barrett (2018) in *How Emotions Are Made*, would go so far as to say that the brain's evolved capacity for linguistic expression has fundamentally altered the networks responsible for interoception—the brain's monitoring and allocation of predicted energy requirements for the body—and, with that, emotion itself as a mechanism proactively managing changing energy needs.

Others would not go so far, but most admit that the language we use and share to name, to express, and to communicate emotions impacts our experience of them. This recognition is central to the burgeoning field of emotions history, as well. If I can distinguish between anger, rage, malice, a grudge, and so on, I can differentiate between those experiences as well, though only to the extent that these words can transact meaning within my socio-cultural group.

As language is so intrinsic to emotional experience, it is no surprise that from antiquity to the present day, people have been using lists as tools for emotional expression and regulation. Paul Ekman gave us six "universal emotions," which he argued are recognizable from facial expressions. His argument, made across multiple works, and the experimental designs underlying it, have been much critiqued, but what remains is the still-current impulse to list—either to modify, expand, or replace his. Of course, long before Ekman, and before William James (1842–1910), early modern philosophers made it a point to include lists of "passions": Thomas Hobbes (1588–1679), Renée Descartes (1596–1650), Baruch Spinoza (1632–1677), among others. All of these sought the "universal" or the "primary" wellsprings of emotion. In antiquity, philosophers and physicians similarly used lists to explore the "primary passions," and, while Plato in the *Timaeus* (69d) and Aristotle in *Rhetoric* 2.1 (1378a20–30), offered somewhat different lists,[4] the Stoic synthesis proved an enduring basis of psychological reflection. They posited four primary, or generic, passions: desire, fear, pleasure, and pain. These marked out humans' impulse toward what preserves life—desire, pleasure—and repulsion from what harms it—fear, pain. Beyond these generic passions, though, Stoics made multiple lists of species, of the various forms these might take. So desire might have five forms, or six, or 13, depending on the list—including terms like eros, yearning, anger, rage, and so on. So too for fear, pleasure, and pain.[5] For example, under "pain," Psuedo-Andronicus (1884) includes the following species:

> Malice is pain at others' blessings, or pain at their deserved successes.
> Envy is pain at another getting one of those things you yourself wanted. Or it is pain at things falling to others but not to us.
> Rivalry is pain at things falling to others, although they fall also to us.
> Misfortune is pain at close-packed sufferings.
> Depression is pain that weighs one down.
> ("On the Passions," 1.2, pp. 12–13)

Pseudo-Andronicus describes species of emotions here in terms of social circumstance (as envy and malice) or bodily sensation (like depression), both of which are important to emotional regimes. Stoic lists thus effectively mediate a top-down approach that begins with psychology and cosmology to explain the mechanisms of emotion, and a bottom-up approach that begins with the myriad experiences of daily life as noted by Graver (2007, p. 57). In their indeterminate length, these lists encouraged further reflection and even addition of emotion-terms. Lists constitute a twofold *technology of emotion*: they organize emotional repertoires and supply language for their expression, a distinction I expand upon in a recent chapter (Zecher, 2023). Christian monastics shared that impulse to list, and in the monastic context developed them into an overarching technology not only of organization and expression, but of transformation through direction.

To the Desert

Cassian, known in the West as John Cassian, and among Eastern Orthodox Christians as Kassianos the Roman, was born around 360 in Roman Dacia—now southern Romania, near the mouth of the Danube. As a young man he travelled south to become a monk at a monastery in Bethlehem. Sometime around 385, he and his friend Germanus were given permission to travel to Egypt, to the heartland of monasticism and the already famous centres of Sketis, Nitria, and Kellia. The two friends would spend years there, but ultimately Cassian was forced to leave Egypt after being enmired in theological controversies. The next few years are shadowy, though we know that he unsuccessfully petitioned the Pope on behalf of John Chrysostom, who had ordained him a deacon. By the 420s he was settled in Gaul and began writing his treatises on monasticism. First, the *Institutes* (420–429), which makes for Gallic monks an exemplar of the form of life found in Egypt—at least, as remembered and interpreted by Cassian. Then, he wrote a series of deeper reflections on the thoughts, emotions, inward dispositions, ultimate aims, and theological conundrums, of monastic spirituality, in the *Conferences* (430), which he completed in three parts, by about 430. In his twilight years, the Pope asked him to write a treatise defending the Incarnation of Christ against Nestorian interpretations. He died sometime around 435.[6]

Cassian's life was too eventful by half. What he wanted was to settle down in Egypt, to live among his heroes and learn from them. One of those, never named among the Abbas of the *Conferences*, was Evagrius of Pontus (c. 345–399), whose disciple Cassian certainly was. Evagrius was a philosopher-cum-monk, who probed the psychological depths of ascetic experience—the thoughts and emotions that beset desert-dwellers were a particular speciality of his. Evagrius was a keen student of experience, to which he added immense philosophical erudition and a keen intellect. So, like the Stoics before him, he made a list of "passions" or, as he put it, "wicked thoughts" or "demons." Here's the order of his list: gluttony, lust, avarice, anger, sadness, acedia, vainglory, and pride.[7] For Evagrius these thoughts—*logismoi*, which might also be rendered "trains of thought"—were a working model of ways in which natural passions and normal emotions become morally blameworthy ones. They are eight generic pathways of dysfunction, meant to include and explain numerous species, just as we saw in Stoic lists. However, with his emphasis on a morally evaluative framework of

Table 2.1 The Eight Thoughts, or Eight Principal Vices of Evagrius and Cassian.

The Eight Thoughts, or Eight Principal Vices		
Evagrius[This is the order]	*Cassian*[8]	*English*
Gastrimargia	*Gastrimargia / Ventris ingluvies*	Gluttony
Porneia	*Fornicatio*	Lust / Fornication
Filarguria	*Filargyria / Avaritia*	Avarice
Orgê	*Ira*	Anger
Lupê	*Tristitia*	Sadness
Akêdia	*Acedia*	Acedia
Kenodoxia	*Cenodoxia / Vana gloria*	Vainglory
Huperêfania	*Superbia*	Pride

demonic temptation and human sin, Evagrius conceived his list more as a diagnostic chart and disciplinary guide for dysfunctional thinking. I offer a fuller discussion of this point in my 2022 work (Zecher, 2022, pp. 128–158).

Note how many of these "thoughts" are clearly emotions: anger, sadness, and acedia—which refers to a kind of anxious boredom, a malaise of the desert—especially. Really, Evagrius would have understood all eight as equally "emotional," because each describes evaluative states with action readiness and affective components. Gluttony is as much "emotional" as anger, and pride as deeply affective as sadness. Evagrius draws emotional states into the moral evaluation of an ascetic, Christian, spirituality, since the eight "thoughts" are as much about dysfunctional motivation as cognition, and it is impossible to disentangle these two modalities.

Cassian took Evagrius's list and ran with it. He not only brought the list into Latin, from which Gregory the Great would later craft the seven deadly sins, but he elaborated Evagrius's working model into the centrepiece of a whole system of spiritual direction. For example, the *Institutes* falls into two parts: Books One to Four cover the prayers, services, dress, and general organization of communal monastic life; Books Five to Twelve are each devoted to one of the eight thoughts. But it is in the *Conferences*, especially the Fifth Conference, with Abba Serapion that Cassian moves from a general assessment of each thought and its counteraction to a deeper analysis of their emergence, manifestation, interrelationships, and development into the lasting defects of character and soul that he calls "vice."

First, Cassian teases out synchronic relationships among the passions. He distinguishes between: those that require some external material—food, money, bodies—and those that do not; those that bring pleasure and those that bring pain; and those that build up and those that tear down. The following table shows these various relations:

Table 2.2 The relations of Cassian's vices to nature, the body, pleasure, and external materials.

Vice	*Come from nature?*	*Require a body?*	*Bring Pleasure?*	*Require something external?*
Gluttony	Yes	Yes	Yes	Yes
Avarice	No	Yes	Yes	Yes
Fornication	Yes	Yes	Yes	Yes
Anger	Yes	No	Yes	Yes
Sadness	Yes	No	No	No
Acedia	Yes	No	No	No
Vainglory	Yes	No	Yes	No
Pride	Yes	No	Yes	No

Most of the vices are natural or, perhaps, exploit the inbuilt passivities and vulnerabilities of human nature. Cassian is adamant, though, that avarice is unnatural, since money and wealth are themselves distortive human inventions. Likewise, most of the passions are about achieving desire for pleasure, or at least for avoiding pain. Anger, though, is a desire born of frustrated desire—a wish for revenge, perhaps. But sadness merely dwells in pain and distress, no longer even seeking a way out, and acedia has almost no direction whatsoever. It is a listlessness without object, a bit like Kierkegaard's *angst* or Baudelaire's *ennui*.[9] There is no pleasure in these. Three vices—gluttony, avarice, and fornication—require a body, but anger too requires external material to be kindled. One can imagine a bodiless mind suffering from pride or anger, as early Christians regularly imagined Satan and the demons to do. But we must assume that, for humans, even non-bodily vices will be worked out in bodily ways and through social relationships. Thoughts and passions pull humans in all different directions, and so the list is also a vector analysis of impulses and motivations. This creates an idea of affinities between those impulses, as well as a sense of what they might need to be counteracted or cured.

Second, Cassian elaborates a dynamic, diachronic, set of relationships, which we can see in the progress of thoughts. He says that each leads to another, and this is in two different ways. First, there is a kind of natural slippage from one to the next. Cassian traces a perhaps surprising line of causation from the pleasure of wealth to the gratification of the stomach and from there to sexual desire and its pleasure. (In antiquity, a rich diet and satiety were thought to arouse sexual thoughts. One purpose of the limited monastic diet was to help quell sexual thoughts. On this topic, see Shaw's 1998 book *The Burden of the Flesh: Fasting and Sexuality in Early Christianity*.) If these desires and pleasures are frustrated, though, anger is aroused; anger frustrated leads to sadness. Sadness prolonged becomes acedia. If, however, someone is able to overcome these first six passions, or to believe they have, then vainglory arises. Vainglory's ultimate form requires no audience and is pride. The movement from the first six passions to vainglory and pride highlights another kind of order, which is defined by monks' own progress in the spiritual life. They likely begin to deal with avarice at the outset, as they renounce personal property, but only later do they deal with acedia, since this experience emerges from the long and isolated routine of a hermit's life. Or, differently, a novice's anger is quite different from an elder's; and vainglory looks different for those who have been ordained and those who remain in the laity. During this process, spiritual direction throws up new thoughts as disciples grow closer to God. Thus, monks must expect to encounter all eight thoughts at various points in their lives, with some being more likely at different stages; but they will encounter them differently as they progress and mature.

Third, there are the lists begotten by this list. Cassian is well aware that the eight primary passions, vices, demonic attacks, have innumerable forms in the moment. These offspring, manifestations, symptoms, are the eight vices as we encounter them in the wild. As did Stoic lists, Cassian strives to connect the experience of the moment with a prior, probably unseen, perhaps unrealized, cause. Sometimes these connections are clear, sometimes counterintuitive. But tracing them is a key part of spiritual direction. The following table gives a sense of the vast array of passions that can emerge, and how Cassian tries to connect them to the eight primary ones. The column on the left is a long, rattling list of vices, which Abba Serapion reels off to Cassian and Germanus. The two columns to the right represent how, in the remainder of his speech, he connects many of those vices to the eight primary ones. A few new ones are introduced, and a few missed out, but we can see how he adapts the technology of the list to explore causation and manifestation:

Table 2.3 Connecting the vices from Abba Serapion's speech to Cassian's eight primary ones.

Conferences 5.26.3	*Conferences 5.26.5*	
...Homicides, arguments, heresies, thefts, false witness, blasphemies, revelry, drunkenness, slanders, jokes, immodest talk, lies, perjuries, drivel, buffoonery, disquiet, rapacity, shouting, indignation, contempt, murmuring, temptation, despair, and many others which it would take too long to list.	Gluttony	revelries, drunkenness
	Lust/Fornication	immodest talk, buffoonery, jokes, drivel
	Avarice	lies, fraud, thefts, perjury, desire for "filthy lucre," false witness, violence, inhumanity, rapacity
	Anger	homicides, shouting, indignation
	Sadness	rancor, pusillanimity, bitterness, despair
	Acedia	hatefulness, sleepiness, importunity, disquiet, wandering, instability of mind and body, verbosity, inappropriate curiosity
	Vainglory	arguments, heresies, ostentation, the presumption of novelty
	Pride	contempt, envy, disobedience, blasphemy, murmuring, slander

Cassian builds on philosophical and earlier monastic traditions to craft an art of emotion. This art relies on the technology of lists which at once organize and articulate a range of emotional experience around core emotions. The lists enable spiritual direction by giving director and disciple a common language and reference. But more than that, they enable interrogation of emotional experience, either to predict where desire may flow next, or to trace the invisible lines backward from manifestation to root cause. This technology, though, is designed for a particular kind of relationship and form of life, presuming an asymmetry of obedience and authority, in which the disciple does not function autonomously. We shall return to this later.

Transformation: From *effectus* to *affectus*

For now, let's pursue the logic of the lists from manifestation to cause. Cassian's lists are not really about what are sometimes called "state" emotions, but about "trait" emotions. Or, in his language, he aims at uncovering and operating on *affectus* [dispositions]. Let's return to the 24th Conference, in which Cassian ties the eight thoughts to the three parts of the Platonic soul: the rational, the spirited/irascible, and the appetitive. Vice, he says, is one and the same, but its emergence differs according to the part of the soul impacted. If the rational, then vice will look like vainglory and pride; if the irascible, then anger, sadness, and acedia; if the appetitive, then gluttony, lust, and avarice. The pathways of dysfunction indicate different locations of damage, different psychic lesions, if you like. The list relies, therefore, on a presumed psychophysical structure of the human being, which the spiritual director must understand, just as a physician must know anatomy.

Let's come back to the different terms Cassian, and Evagrius before him, use: thoughts, demons, passions, and vices. Each term indexes some aspect of embodiment, passivity, and character formation. Thoughts emerge quickly, perhaps sporadically. They are episodic, giving rise to momentary "state emotions." But as these thoughts are indulged, they become dispositional, and "state emotions" become "trait emotions," part of the disposition. Cassian reserves language of "vice" to describe what happens when particular emotional dysfunctions have oozed through a person's whole character. For example, anger is a passion but is only called a vice when we are talking about an "angry person." This may or may not erupt in rages or abusive language, but it persists beneath the surface. His regular references to demons remind us that, for Cassian, humans inhabit a world filled with other minds, some benevolent, many malevolent. Since he maps the possible dysfunctions of emotion and cognition, it is also a list of human vulnerabilities to outside, demonic, attack and exploitation. (He discusses demonic attack and temptation especially in *Conferences*, 7–8.) Thus, whether roused by an old memory, a fresh incident, or a more inexplicable and intrusive thought, Cassian believes that we go awry in these eight ways. Cassian's discipline of emotions through lists cannot be understood apart from a cosmology in which demons, angels, and monks cohabitate the desert, and in which affective disposition is decisive for a person's character.

Cassian's spiritual direction drills down to those underlying dispositions while appreciating the ecosystem of thoughts, demons, and so on. Thus, he has Abba John lament in the 19th Conference that "When, therefore, we notice signs of vices in our heart, we know clearly that we do not lack the disposition to sin, but only its action" (*Conferences*, 19.12.4). Or elsewhere, Cassian says that people like Job are praised and Judas Iscariot blamed not just for their actions, but for the dispositions in accordance with which they acted (*Conferences*, 6.9.1). If we read this in light of Cassian's various lists, we can understand that he offers readers ways to relate state emotions back to trait emotions—the numerous offspring of anger are all the effects of an angry disposition; the various species of avarice are ways that habit comes to action; and so on. Spiritual direction operates not so much on the offspring as on their often-invisible cause.

To Values

There is a popular myth that Stoics—and, like them, early Christians—aimed to rid themselves of emotion. There is some truth in the claim that Stoics aimed for "apatheia" by which they meant a tranquillity impervious to strong emotional shocks. But in fact, theologians like Cassian were concerned not with extirpating emotions but with correcting and training them. They did not seek the cessation of desire, but a rightly directed one.

Let's go back to Germanus and Cassian's confession. Their thoughts of homesickness actually included three different motives: first, they imagine themselves comforted and supported by family members; second, they imagine themselves guiding their family to salvation; third, they dwell on the beauty and bounty of their homeland—a stark contrast to the brutality of the Egyptian desert. Abba Abraham sees in these three motivations attachments and values at odds with the monastic life. Primary is the desire for comfort, which requires material and familial support. But the idea of leading family to salvation, which seems good on its face, in fact shows the brothers to be suffering from vainglory: a misplaced desire for glory and a mis-cognition of their own status. Their homesickness results, in fact, from misplaced values and perceptions, of themselves and their families.

The values that people hold dear are the glue for their emotional dispositions. This means that, when Cassian operates on those dispositions, he does so by attacking the values that hold them together, as we see with Abba Abraham. Spiritual direction works at exposing those values and attachments. In service of this, the eight thoughts are an index of mistaken or malicious values, in relation to one's environment, one's body, one's status, and one's self-image. Each thought marks a field of dysfunction based on mis-valuation and, with it, mis-cognition. But the change of disposition sought after must rest on a new valuation, a new cognition—and that comes with a new form of life. This new form of life does not reject emotions but entails even stronger ones. Thus, in his discussion of chastity, Cassian says of sexual desire:

> Desires for things present could not be restrained or removed unless, in place of these harmful emotional dispositions—which we yearn to have amputated—other, salubrious ones were introduced. For in no other way is the mind's vivacity able to subsist, save by the affect of some desire or fear, joy or grief.
>
> (*Conferences*, 12.5.3)

Spiritual direction comprises a transplant operation, with the director working surgically on emotional dispositions and the values that underpin them. The goal is not an extirpation of emotion or of desire, but a return to their proper object and operation. In the story with which I opened this chapter, Abba Abraham chides Cassian and Germanus for their *lack of ardor, their lack of desire.* The remedies he offers centre on focusing their emotional regime around a totalizing desire for God that can only be achieved through the monastic form of life.

Cassian's list is explicitly diagnostic, and it carries with it a therapeutic alternative: the development of what Cassian calls "healthy dispositions." Since dispositions are built up through long periods of habituation, spiritual direction is ongoing as well as interventive. Cassian imagines a life-long process within this relationship, with confession at its heart: to open up not just actions but thoughts, ideas, plans, feelings, momentary distractions, whatever one is experiencing, to the scrutiny and interpretation of one's elder. Cassian describes doing just this with Abba Moses (*Conferences*, 2.10.1–3). On the basis of that confession, the elder assigns homework. Discipline and penance, but also more generally targeted practices of psalmody, recitation, labor, eschatological meditation, and so on. (Cassian discusses the more practical matters of monastic life in *Institutes* 1–4, with remedies for individual vices in the remaining books.) For Cassian as for others, reciting the Psalms is so central to monastic practice and so frequently advised by directors because, more than anything else, the Psalms were thought to operate on emotional dispositions. Cassian says that, through repeated chanting, "a monk receives in himself all the dispositions of the Psalms" (*Conferences*, 10.11.4). The Psalms provide a new emotional repertoire, including both language and scripts for expressing healthy emotions and rejecting sinful ones. In turn, these meditative, recitative, and mnemonic strategies, including recitation of the Psalms, are bolstered by regular confession not just of sins, but of thoughts as they occur, of dreams, and of memories. The process of spiritual direction operates on a dialectic of confession and discipline aimed at transforming dispositions.

As technologies, lists are both diagnostic and normative, allowing disciples and their abbas to make sense of a bewildering array of emotions and to relate them to a stable causal framework. At the same time, Cassian's program of emotional direction is basically therapeutic, aimed at reconfiguring the monk's disposition, understood within the framework of thoughts and vices. Spiritual direction's emphasis on dispositions points us back to the "form of life" which monastics aimed at. Here we have the core of spiritual direction as a transformative process. To borrow Nietzsche's (2022 [1887], p. 16) phrase from *The Genealogy of Morals*, spiritual direction is a "revaluation of all values" which takes place within a totalizing relationship, one that embraces and makes demands on every part of the disciple's life. In this revaluation, tools like the eight vices provide for the articulation of dysfunction but, more than that, transformation and healing in each area. Cassian aims at transformation, rather than the extirpation, of emotion—so that the path to vice and the path to virtue both run through the emotional landscape of desire. The end and aim of these practices are prayer, by which Cassian would have understood union and conversation of the intellect with God. He puts it another way in the First Conference: the monk's end is the Kingdom of Heaven, but they arrive there only through *puritas cordis* [purity of heart]. Purity of heart means, for Cassian, tranquillity and chastity, a fully healthy disposition built on right values, right attachments, right perceptions, attained and maintained through desire.

The Challenges of Values

Cassian is explicit: spiritual direction in the monastic life is about healing. He presumes that the monk begins sick, "sick with desire/ And fastened to a dying animal" as Yeats (1933) says in "Sailing to Byzantium" (stanza III). This sickness requires diagnosis, for which lists provide the technology and confession the opportunity. The practices and rhythms of monastic life provide therapies targeted to particular kinds of emotion, to particular parts of the soul, and conducive to particular virtues. For him, spiritual direction is clinical in the deepest sense of the word and transformative in the long term.

So, this raises questions as we think about spiritual direction in context of other modes of therapy, analysis, and clinical situations. Cassian—and with him many other Christian monastic thinkers (enough, indeed, that I might call them a tradition)—lays a claim both to spiritual direction *and* to clinical care. For him these are not distinct, and they cannot be distinct, in part because the disease is sin and its cure an ascetic—probably monastic—form of life. But that kind of claim presents challenges as we reflect on plural modes of spiritual direction and secular or, at least, deliberately de-traditionalized forms. It presents further complications as we consider the right relationship, the overlap or difference between spiritual direction and therapies.

The "self" created is a self that is suited for a particular kind of life and community. Cassian's "self" is a harmony of interlocking parts—the parts of the soul, the organs and members of the body. It is also part of an ecosystem including inanimate, vegetable, animal, human, and non-human minds. If we take seriously the monastic language of demons and angels, the human being formed through practices of spiritual direction must interact with and be impacted by these other minds. More generally, the values and emotional dispositions for which Cassian aims make sense within certain conditions—but these are as limited as they are profound. The conditions are defined by adherence to a faith, a tradition, and a concrete community. Can we, then, speak of common aims in spiritual direction across different traditions, communities, and faiths? Or must the aims be specific and plural? Does plurality mean irreducible difference, or are we better off looking for common ground in spiritual direction?

That community and its membership raises further questions also of autonomy and dependence. The form of life Cassian inscribes into his *Conferences* presumes that the human being is a certain kind of thing, a porous and embedded collection of parts that should operate in certain configurations. The work of spiritual direction draws the human toward what they are meant to be and, in that regard, closer to God. But the normative assumptions underlying this cannot be ignored. Thus, while I've focused on the individual relationship of director and disciple, Cassian is clear that directors hand on the wisdom of their elders, and the practices of their community formed across multiple generations (*Conferences*, 2.13.2). Thus, the individual relationship has a genealogy that is frequently invisible. Can that relationship be imagined without the tradition and community behind it? Or is that a different *kind* of thing altogether? This in turn raises the question of extracting and applying monastic wisdom outside of monastic communities. How can these relationships be translated, constituted, and configured for laypeople, for those in different religious traditions, for those seeking direction without affiliation?

And then there is the mode of relationship. Cassian thinks hierarchically: the director not only leads the disciple but acts as arbiter of their thoughts and feelings, and as judge of their progress. This kind of authoritarianism puts Cassian at odds with articulations of spiritual direction as companionship. It certainly sets Cassian at odds with that neoliberal individualism and autonomy which so many of us cherish. But perhaps there is value in thinking through hierarchy—so long as it is checked. For Cassian, it is the community that checks the authority of an individual elder, and tradition that checks the community—and God that gives tradition. The relationship between elder and disciple can only make sense within that transpersonal and transhistorical web of relationships that create mutuality within hierarchy. This, if nothing else, is a valuable reminder to ask what sort of community or communities contextualize spiritual direction today? How are individual relationships conceived and cared for?

Finally, I have mentioned emotional "regimes" a few times in connection with the aims of spiritual direction. Emotional transformation presumes a norm or ideal of emotional regulation. Cassian's writings do not leave much room for divergent emotional "styles." Rather, they enforce "regimes"—normative patterns of emotion based on moral and social evaluations, which are in turn enforced through group pressure. The network of relationships and the form of life which underpin monastic spiritual direction have a strong disciplinary dimension. Michel Foucault, when writing on Cassian, saw this as a deliberate self-annihilation through obedience.[10] I think that's basically incorrect, because submission is itself a focalization and intensification of the will and desire, but it does seem clear that for monastics, submitting to spiritual direction means submitting to a process of discipline and formation in which individual autonomy is often punished as refusal of the normative ideal.

On one level, of course, these texts are simply being honest about how emotional styles work within communities. Sociologists and psychologists have long understood emotions as having scripts—indeed, being scripted. These scripts are written and determined in advance through social interactions frequently unchosen or unrealized. Cassian's lists and the authority of the director simply expose those scripts for what they are.

But there is a pernicious side to lists. Lists discipline by pathologizing. Are Cassian's lists totally different from the syndromal lists of the DSM-5-TR, or ICD-11 codes? Are they, in fact, ways of pathologizing difference? Or is there a space within the impulse to list to attend to difference as well as norms, to discover and cherish this person precisely as a person—not an individual, but their own web of relations, histories, aims, and aspirations?

With these questions in mind, I hope that Cassian and, with him, the early Christian monastic tradition which he represents and, through Benedict and others, helped found, offers fresh ways of thinking about the centrality of emotional experience and transformation in spiritual direction. I hope also that his unblinking commitment to traditions, norms, and hierarchies can challenge us as we consider the values that underpin spiritual direction and the values that spiritual direction itself challenges.

Notes

1 All translations are my own and refer to the critical edition by Michael Petschenig: *Cassiani opera. Collationes XXIIII*, (Cassian, 1888). However, for those interested in reading Cassian further, Boniface Ramsey, OSB has produced marvellous translations of both the *Conferences* (Cassian, 1997 [430]) and *Institutes* (Cassian, 1998 [420–429]).

2 While emotional theorists may share this nomenclature with "affect theory," I am not talking about the kind of undifferentiated intensity associated with affect theorists like Deleuze and Guattari or Brian Massumi. With emotions we are talking about cognitive phenomena, inseparable from linguistic reflection, even if beginning in pre-cognitive domains. Of course, some scientists lead us to wonder if there

are such pre-cognitive phenomena, or if even the neurological basis of emotions is, in a sense, cognitive (e.g. Barrett and Russell, 2014; and Barrett, 2018).

3 [Aristotle], *Problemata* 2026 (569a5–6) = Basil of Caesarea (?), *Commentary on Isaiah* 5.181 (PG 30:424A), Dorotheos of Gaza, *Instructions* 8, in Dorotheos of Gaza, *Discourses and Sayings*, trans. Eric Wheeler, Cistercian Studies 33 (Kalamazoo: Cistercian Publications, 1977), 150.

4 In the *Timaeus* (69d) and *Rhetoric* 2.1 (1378a20–30), respectively.

5 Key Stoic lists are found in Arius Didymus, *Epitome of Stoic Ethics*; Ps-Andronicus of Rhodes, *On the Passions*; Diogenes Laertius, *Lives of the Philosophers* 7.113–116. These were Christianized by Nemesius of Emesa (4th c.), in his *On Human Nature* 17–21, and his version became the standard for Maximus the Confessor (7th) and John of Damascus (8th) in the Christian East, and later for Thomas Aquinas (13th), among others in the West. The Stoic lists have, therefore, a long history of organizing emotion and early modern philosophers crafted their lists of primary passions partly in response to this tradition.

6 There are several excellent introductions to Cassian's life and thought, though the work of Columba Stewart, OSB, Cassian the Monk (1998), is probably the best starting point, but see also Steven Driver's *John Cassian and the Reading of Egyptian Monastic Culture* (2002) and more recently Niki Kasumi Clements's *Sites of the Ascetic Self: John Cassian and Christian Ethical Formation* (2020).

7 Evagrius discusses the eight in the *Praktikos, On the Eight Thoughts, The Eight Spirits of Wickedness, The Virtues Opposed to the Vices*, and *On Thoughts*, all of which are accessible in Robert Sinkewicz's *Evagrius of Pontus. The Greek Ascetic Corpus* (Sinkewicz, 2003).

Evagrius uses in *On the Eight Spirits of Wickedness*, see Sinkewicz (2003). In other texts, like *Vices Opposed to Virtues*, he transposes anger and sadness.

8 I take this version from *Conferences* 5.2.

9 Soren Kierkegaard, *The Concept of Anxiety: A Simple Psychologically Orienting Deliberation on the Dogmatic Issue of Hereditary Sin*, ed. and trans. Reidar Thomte with Albert B. Anderson, Kierkegaard's *Writings* 8 (Princeton, NJ: Princeton University Press, 1980); Charles Baudelaire, "*Au Lecteur* [To the Reader]," in Charles Baudelair, *The Flowers of Evil.* With Parallel French Text, trans. James McGowan, Oxford World Classics (Oxford: OUP, 1998), 4–7.

10 Michel Foucault, "The Battle for Chastity", in Philippe Ariès and André Béjin (eds), *Western Sexuality: Practice and Precept in Past and Present Times*, trans. Anthony Forster (New York: Blackwell, 1985), 14–25. He offers a more sympathetic analysis of Christian spiritual direction, although with regard to a different set of authors, in *History of Sexuality*, vol. 4: *Confessions of the Flesh*, ed. Frédéric Gros, trans. Robert Hurley (New York: Vintage Books, 2021).

References

Barrett, L. F. and Russell, J. A. (Eds.). (2014). *The Psychological Construction of Emotion*. Guildford Press.

Barrett, L. F. (2018). *How Emotions are Made: The Secret Life of the Brain*. Harper.

Cassian, J. (1888). *Cassiani opera Collationes* XXIIII (M. Petschenig, Ed.). Christianorum

Scriptorum Ecclesiasticorum Latinorum 13.

Cassian, J. (1997). *The Conferences* (B. Ramsey, Trans.). Ancient Christian Writers 57.

Newman Press. (Original text completed c. 430.)

Cassian, J. (1998). *The Institutes* (B. Ramsey, Trans.). Ancient Christian Writers 58. Newman

Press. (Original text written 420–429.)

Champion, M. W., Garrod, R., Haskell, Y., and Ruys, J. (2019). But were they talking about the emotions? Affectus, affectio and the history of emotions. *Rivista Storica Italiana*, 128, 521–543.

Clements, N. K. (2020). *Sites of the Ascetic Self: John Cassian and Christian Ethical Formation*. University of Notre Dame Press.

Driver, S. (2002). *John Cassian and the Reading of Egyptian Monastic Culture.* Routledge.

Frijda, N. H. (1986). *The Emotions.* Cambridge University Press.

Frijda, N. H. (2006). *The Laws of Emotion.* Taylor and Francis.

Frijda, N. H. (2016). *The evolutionary emergence of what we call "emotions." Cognition and Emotion*, 30, 609–620.

Graver, M. (2007). *Stoicism and Emotion.* University of Chicago Press.

Laertius, D. (1925). *Lives of the Philosophers* (R. W. Hicks, Trans.). Loeb Classical Library. Harvard University Press.

Mesquita, B. (2022). *Between Us: How Cultures Create Emotion.* Norton.

Nietzsche, F. (2022). *The Genealogy of Morals* (T. Newcomb, Trans.). Newcomb Livraria Press. (Original work published 1887.)

Nussbaum, M. (2001). *Upheavals of Thought: The Intelligence of Emotions.* Cambridge University Press.

Pseudo-Andronicus. (1884). On the Passions, in X. Kreuttner (Ed.), *Andronici qui fertur libelli Περί παθῶν (De affectibus), Pars Prior: De passionibus.* Winter.

Reddy, W. F. (2001). *The Navigation of Feeling: A Framework for the History of Emotions.* Cambridge University Press.

Scarantino, A. (2014). The Motivational Theory of Emotions. In J. D'Arms and D. Jacobson (Eds.), *Moral Psychology and Human Agency: Philosophical Essays on the Science of Ethics.* (pp. 156–185). Oxford University Press.

Scheer, M. (2012). Are emotions a kind of practice (and is that what makes them have a history)? A Bourdieuian approach to understanding emotion. *History and Theory*, 51193–220.

Shaw, T. M. (1998). *The Burden of the Flesh: Fasting and Sexuality in Early Christianity.* Fortress.

Sinkewicz, R. (2003). *Evagrius of Pontus. The Greek Ascetic Corpus.* Oxford Early Christian Studies. Oxford University Press.

Solomon, R. (1976). *The Passions: Emotions and the Meaning of Life.* Doubleday.

Stewart, C. (1998). *Cassian the Monk.* Oxford University Press.

Tappolet, C. (2016). *Emotions, Values, and Agency.* Oxford University Press.

Yeats, W. B. (1933). *The Poems of W. B. Yeats: A New Edition* (R. J. Finneran, Ed.). Macmillan Publishing Company.

Zecher, J. L. (2022). *Spiritual Direction as a Medical Art in Early Christian Monasticism.* Oxford Early Christian Studies. Oxford University Press.

Zecher, J. L. (2023). Affective lexica between Hellenistic philosophy and Christian theology. In J. R. Clarke, D. King, and H. Baltussen (Eds.), *Pain Narratives in Greco-Roman Writings: Studies in the Representation of Physical and Mental Suffering*. (pp. 273–298). Studies in Ancient Medicine, 58. Brill.

Chapter 3

Psychoanalysis in the House of Ignatius and the New Age

Pamela Cooper-White

C. G. Jung on several occasions compared Ignatius of Loyola's (1999 [1522–1524]) *Spiritual Exercises* (1522–1524) to analytical psychology—his version of psychoanalysis—especially regarding the maturational process he termed "individuation," stating that the *Exercises* constituted "a serious business that takes hold of people at the deepest level" (Jung, 2023 [1939–1940], p. 189). In this chapter, I propose to examine this claim by addressing several questions. First, what is spiritual direction? The practice has, after all, expanded well beyond the ever-growing Ignatian Christian model (e.g., Fleming, 2016; Ganss, 1991; Harter, 2005), including a proliferation of forms drawing from multiple indigenous and non-Western religious traditions and/or loosely fitting under the umbrella of "New Age." Second, where does spiritual direction overlap with psychotherapy—much less psychoanalysis? How is it distinctively different, and where are appropriate boundaries? Third, how can psychoanalytic perspectives and insights—judiciously applied—possibly enrich the practice of spiritual direction without taking a clinical-therapeutic turn? As there are as many branches of psychoanalysis as there are now modes of spiritual direction, this portion of the paper will open what can only be a preliminary discussion regarding both potential resources and pitfalls for spiritual direction relating to Jung, Winnicott, Kohut, and contemporary relational psychoanalysis.[1] Of course, one cannot neglect Freud and European psychoanalysis, especially prior to the importing of a rigidified "classical psychoanalysis" (i.e., ego psychology) to the US by the émigré analysts during WWII and the Holocaust (Kuriloff, 2013). Will there also be a mention of Lacan? Wait and see…

What Is Spiritual Direction Today?

First, what is spiritual direction? The term itself has been adopted far beyond its origins in Ignatian and other Catholic, Orthodox, and Anglican traditions. There is a large and growing literature on this subject, not to mention the proliferation of conferences, workshops, and retreats led by organizations such as Spiritual Directors International (SDI, n.d.)[2] and an increasing number of training programs—offered by both accredited graduate schools

DOI: 10.4324/9781003742852-3

and unaccredited organizations.[3] The underlying theologies, cosmologies, and cultural origins of the many forms of spiritual direction—including other terms such as "spiritual companionship"—differ greatly. Some root firmly in a particular religious or spiritual tradition—such as pre-modern Celtic spirituality, Christian monasticism and related contemplative traditions, Jewish mysticism, and Eastern traditions such as Buddhism. Other forms are more eclectic, drawing from a variety of traditions—at best, in respectful ways, and at worst, as a smorgasbord of cultural appropriation. Even the terms "direction" and "director" are contested as being too hierarchical, but alternatives fall short of describing the differing roles of "director" and "directee"—especially when payment and fiduciary responsibility of the director are involved.

Of course, the term "spiritual"—or "spirituality"—is an even bigger problematic, seeming to encompass almost anything that an individual or group might subjectively identify as such. As spirituality became more a field of study in the 1980s and beyond, the Psychology, Culture, and Religion group of the American Academy of Religion became a locus for sometimes heated discussions about the many meanings and uses of the term. The group also facilitated critiquing both the looseness of spirituality's definitions and the ways in which personalized rituals replicate but do not acknowledge or are shorn from the traditional roots and cultures from which they have been reinvented or stolen without attribution (e.g., Bregman, 2014).

Following Paul Tillich's (1957) definition of "faith," I will likewise extend his definition to apply also to the "spiritual" as that which has to do with matters of "ultimate concern." Given the wide variety of religious and spiritual traditions and pathways found among seekers of spiritual direction today, I believe Tillich's definition still has both the breadth and depth to stand the test of time. Tillich's definition of pastoral care in his address to a very early meeting of the National Conference of Clinical Pastoral Education in 1958 is similarly relevant today: "a helping encounter in the dimension of ultimate concern" (Tillich, 1959, p. 22). This definition may be even more relevant and more widely accepted today, as the whole field of pastoral and spiritual care—with its longstanding embeddedness in Protestant Christian theology and helping paradigms—is now being challenged by the need for a much wider inter-religious and intercultural approach. For example, in the shift in nomenclature from "pastoral care" to "spiritual care" in medical and nursing departments, hospitals, prisons, and military chaplaincy, we see both Tillich's definition and method—grounded in his own Pauline and Lutheran tradition and in "the Christian message," but even more deeply grounded in the ineffable, the Unconditional, the Ground of Being from which all religious and spiritual traditions mysteriously arise (Cooper-White, 2021, p. 212).

As Tillich was very much influenced by the existentialist movement in 20th-century Europe, we might also understand ultimate concern as having to do with the "big questions" of life and death, meaning and purpose.

Following that line of thinking, I would then describe "spiritual direction" as a relationship in which one person offers a safe space for another person to explore those big questions. If it is to be done well, I also assume that a "spiritual director" is someone who has gone through such a process themselves. I think of this as someone who is on a similar path of spiritual exploration, but further along and acquainted with both the fruits and the perils of such a journey—and as a "director" who has also done some significant training with more experienced directors and supervisors.

How Do Spiritual Direction and Psychotherapy/Psychoanalysis Differ, and Where Are the Boundaries?

So how is this different from providing spiritual or pastoral care or pastoral psychotherapy, or even a very exploratory form of analysis such as the Jungian process of assisting a person in the maturational process of individuation? Thomas Hart, who is both a spiritual director and a psychologist, wrote in the spiritual direction journal *Presence* in 2005 that ultimately, although therapy and spiritual direction normally involve different contexts and training, there is considerable overlap because, in his words (to a couple who came to him for marital counseling), "at bottom all issues are spiritual… I mean that they have to do with the kinds of persons you are making of yourselves" (Hart, 2005, p. 11). In both practices, he notes, the quality of relationship is key. It is a relationship in which the client would say:

> I feel safe with you. I know you care for me. I can talk freely about anything. You listen respectfully and carefully. You are wise and gentle, yet honest with me. I know you believe in me and have hope for me. And the perspectives, suggestions, and support you give are usually very helpful.
> (p. 11)

Hart names honesty and being attentive to the practitioner's own feelings as key to both therapy and direction. His main point is that "although there are four distinguishable types of helping professionals [psychotherapists, pastoral counselors, 'ordinary pastors,' and spiritual directors], there is considerable overlap among them. Psychology and spirituality are easily blended, in various proportions and various ways, across the spectrum" (p. 12).

So what really is the difference? I would say the main difference is in the stated aim and focus. The aim of therapy—including pastoral counseling, psychotherapy, and psychoanalysis—is to address something that is causing the patient or client unease or distress. This is not to say that a person might not seek out spiritual direction because of a perceived spiritual or existential dis-ease. But that is where the focus—*how* one takes up this dis-ease—is especially important. In counseling, the focus is more on problem-solving. In therapy, the focus is on the client or patient. More specifically, in psychotherapy and especially psychoanalysis, the focus is increasingly on what insight can be gleaned about the patient's self-defeating unconscious dynamics from examining the relationship between the therapist and the patient themselves—that is, the transference–countertransference relationship and what it may be re-enacting from the patient's early childhood and subsequent traumas. On the spectrum from counseling to therapy to analysis, however, the focus remains on the client or patient and their troubles, including mental health challenges. Existential therapist Irvin Yalom (1989) once wrote that his usual first question on meeting a new patient is "What ails?" (p. 232). The presumption—and the invitation—is to explore fearlessly the sources of disease a patient is experiencing, in the service of healing and greater wholeness. With or without reference to the *DSM* (American Psychiatric Association, 2022), and whether they—or we—like it or not, most therapists are trained to think in terms of pathology as defined by the medical establishment. This has been disputed and even rejected outright by many pastoral counselors and other strength-based models of counseling for decades. Yet as a way of creating a treatment plan, a diagnostic formulation can be extremely helpful, as long as it doesn't set up assumptions that deny the patient's actual complexity, their healthy parts, and sources of strength (Cooper-White, 2012).

In spiritual direction, by contrast, the focus is not on the client's or directee's problems or pathology. Nor is the focus on the relationship—especially in its unconscious dynamics—between the director and the directee, except if that relationship becomes problematic at certain points and needs to be managed. The focus is not really on the client at all, but rather the focus of both director and directee is a collaborative focus on G-d, the divine, the sacred, or at its most secular, the existential meaning(s) that the directee is seeking to make of their life and its purpose. Often this focus centers around a discernment of vocation or sense of calling. The initial motivation is not "what ails"—unless the dis-ease is specifically a sense of spiritual lack or struggle; but rather, to quote "The Summer Day" by poet Mary Oliver (1990), "what is it you plan to do/ with your one wild and precious life?" (p. 60). And the work is, together, to trace the movement, the patterns, the footprints of Spirit in their life, and how it might be beckoning them toward something new. Pastoral theologian Norma Wood puts it even more succinctly: "*The Holy Spirit is understood to be the Director*, and guidance is mediated by one who listens to another's interior world and guides [them] through prayer, meditation, and discernment of God's leading presence in [their] life" (Wood, 2020, p. 113, emphasis added).

I once attended a workshop for pastoral counselors led by Tilden Edwards of the Shalem Institute.[4] He observed that in our work as therapists, we tend to lean forward toward the client. He asked us to listen to a partner while leaning back instead, shifting our focus toward where we sense the Spirit moving in, around, and between us. We then talked about how different that felt, and how much it opened up for both partners.

Of course, in actuality, Hart (2005) is correct, that the spiritual and the psychological cannot be so neatly separated, and that the directee's life, relationships, and problems cannot be cordoned off from spiritual seeking. But the focus of spiritual direction is on "where is G-d/Spirit/the sacred in all of this?" If pathology does appear as a roadblock to the directee's spiritual growth—and by this I mean real evidence of mental illness or addiction—the proper response of a spiritual director is to refer to a therapist or addiction counselor. For this reason, among many, peer supervision and consultation are core values of Spiritual Director International. Psychotherapists, likewise, who do not have any kind of religious or spiritual training, might be equally well advised to acknowledge a patient's spiritual struggles as part of the human condition, but not to take over the role of spiritual director.

Should a person be in both direction and therapy at the same time? That is a messy question. The main danger is that such a division between the spiritual care and the psychological treatment can create a split in the transference that doesn't serve either practice best. Important revelations may be made in one setting but not the other, leaving both practitioners in the dark about some of the client's most pressing inner concerns. Spiritual directors may invite in more psychological content, believing that it is already being "handled" by the therapist, while the therapist may shunt off to the director certain spiritual concerns that could actually be relevant to the patient's distress. Both practitioners may end up with only a partial understanding of the client, leading to misunderstandings, even impasses.

The patient/client may also unconsciously split the transference into "good helper" and "bad helper," or any number of other possible psychic divisions based on the client's own internal object world. These enactments cannot be easily interpreted by the therapist because they happen, at least in part, elsewhere. Meanwhile, such meaning-laden enactments may pass without notice by the spiritual director who is not trained to work psychoanalytically in the transference, and in whose role such exploration or interpretation of transferential dynamics should not be attempted—even when the director is also a therapist. It's not the same "contract." When a director does notice something that seems to fall outside the norms of that particular directee's work, the appropriate response is to hold it, ponder its meaning, and allow it to help shape the directee's next responses—even perhaps in another session—or to note a flag signaling the need for the client to move into psychotherapy with another appropriate practitioner.

(How) Can Psychoanalysis Benefit Spiritual Direction?

Having set apart the practices of psychotherapy and psychoanalysis from spiritual direction, can spiritual directors still benefit from some of the insights of psychoanalysis, without trying to become pseudo-analysts? Of course, the short and simple answer is that all spiritual directors would benefit from having undergone psychotherapy or analysis themselves—in the main, so that they would become aware of their countertransference and not let unresolved personal or psychological issues interfere with their capacity to understand the directee (Cooper-White, 2004, 2007). More will be said about that below. But beyond this, are there additional aspects of psychoanalytic theory and attunement that can benefit the practice of spiritual direction?

Psychoanalytic Attention to the Third

Therapy is usually thought of as dyadic, focusing on the relationship between analyst and patient (i.e., the transference–countertransference continuum) whereas spiritual direction is triadic, with both director and directee focused on G-d as a third—or even leading—partner. However, to complicate matters further, relational psychoanalysis, because of its emphasis on intersubjectivity[5] and unconscious relationship, also invokes a "Third." Although Jessica Benjamin (2017) and Thomas Ogden (2004) would define this Third somewhat differently, we might boil this down to say that the Third is the relationship itself, or rather, a third subjectivity that is the relationship itself, mostly unconscious, mostly manifested in enactments. When impasses occur, the analysis focuses on this Third, and what it might be "saying" to both analyst and analysand about what is going on in the unconscious flow of relationship between them. This understanding of Third is not the same thing as G-d or Spirit; it remains in the interpersonal realm, not the *trans*-personal.

Jungian analysts, however, would make an exception to that stance if it is perceived that an archetype is doing the enacting from within the patient or the therapeutic dyad. Moreover, these archetypes lead to the collective unconscious and—in transpersonal therapy—to the divine beyond Self. This is where some forms of Jungian analysis may overlap quite a bit with spiritual direction. A Jungian approach to dreamwork has also been incorporated by some—now classic—writers on spiritual direction (e.g., Sanford, 1989; Kelsey, 1978). There is a vast literature on Jung and spirituality, which cannot be summarized within the scope of this paper. (For a good recent discussion pertaining directly to depth psychology and spiritual direction, see Ensign, 2023.)

Increasing Attention to Social Context Beyond the Consulting Room

But how might psychoanalysis that did *not* split off into Jung's analytical psychology still be of help in spiritual direction—even with its inheritance of Freud's atheism? Here, too, there is a vast literature on Freud and religion (summarized, e.g., in Cooper-White, 2018). We could, of course, rehearse the Swiss analyst-pastor Oskar Pfister's (1993 [1928]) rejoinder to Freud's objections about religious faith, and Pfister's own practice of a liberative pastoral psychotherapy utilizing Freud's theory and technique (Cooper-White, 2018, pp. 93–124; Noth and Morgenthaler, 2014). Additionally, we might query, as pastoral theologian Duane Bidwell did in his doctoral dissertation and in an article for the *Journal of Pastoral Theology* (Bidwell, 2003, 2004), the overall tendency of spiritual direction to draw theory and practice from the psychodynamic and depth psychologies of the early 20th century. Bidwell counters this by suggesting social constructionism—a form of social psychology—as another useful resource, especially citing the works of Kenneth J. Gergen (e.g., Gergen, 1999). There is much in social constructionism and especially constructivism—a theory of co-constructed reality—that aligns well with the relational psychoanalytic emphasis on intersubjectivity, especially in practice as Bidwell describes.

The concern for context and social justice had just begun to break through robustly in the field of pastoral theology by the early 1990s, beginning with such texts as Couture (1991) and Graham (1992), summarized in Ramsay (2018). The turn from focusing on psychology and clinical treatment toward care for persons and groups caught up in social injustice has continued with an increasingly diverse group of authors, especially in the Society for Pastoral Theology (SPT, n.d.).[6]

Psychoanalysts themselves also began to take up this critique (e.g., Altman 2009; Belkin and White, 2020; Cushman, 1995; Layton, 2020).[7] Others have done so in querying the lack of attention to social and political context in psychoanalysis—recovering the social reform dimensions of psychoanalysis in Europe in the 1920s by such important early figures as Anna Freud and Otto Fenichel (Jacoby, 1983; Kuriloff, 2013). In the early 1960s, Frantz Fanon was also introducing his revolutionary postcolonial work, using Freud's writings and psychoanalysis as one lens to understand the dynamics of racial systems of oppression, and their impact on persons of color (e.g., Fanon, 2021 [1952], 2004 [1961]).

Recommendations from Freud and Contemporary Relational Psychoanalysis

All psychoanalytic schools of thought are founded in Freud's insistence that there is an unconscious! That much is obvious. But in my experience, many spiritual directors simply don't think about the unconscious very much, or if they do, they try to avoid dealing with it directly, perceiving it as treading too far into the realm of psychotherapy. I'm not talking about encouraging spiritual directors to now begin to interpret unconscious motivations of their directees, much less interpreting the transference. But I would urge spiritual directors—just as I do spiritual and pastoral caregivers—to be aware that there is always more going on with a directee than what appears on the surface. I have three recommendations gleaned from Freudian analysis:

1 Listen with what Theodor Reik (1948) called a "third ear"—a register of paying attention to the gaps and nonverbal communications—for what might be going on with a directee that is not being shared aloud. Not to interpret it, or even name it—that should be the domain of a therapist;

but to be alert to areas of dis-ease, even spiritual dis-ease, that cannot yet be spoken. Then simply hold this awareness lightly, tentatively—we could be wrong of course; and therefore be open to what might emerge down the road. Especially from one theory within relational psychoanalysis, we can also consider that we all contain worlds, we are all multiple subjectivities, we are all multiple.[8] So, the self—sometimes thought of as the present self- or affect-state—that is presenting to the director right now is one *part* of the directee, and other selves may yet appear and bring other spiritual questions, concerns, or struggles. Further, different parts of the directee's self may also be relating to different Gods or God-imagoes (Cataldo, 2008)!

2 Recognize that what's coming up in us as we listen may be our own classical countertransference (described in detail in Cooper-White, 2004). These may be our own unresolved issues, our own "baggage" that can get in the way of fully hearing the other, and we need to take responsibility for this on our own time and sort it out so that we can listen more clearly to the directee. Nevertheless, through the intersubjective shared space of the unconscious relationship—what we are feeling, thinking, fantasizing, experiencing in the relationship—there might also be a hint of something that is coming up in the directee that they cannot voice. A therapist or analyst would likely hold this and wait a while to see if it emerges on its own, or if the feeling "ripens" over some period of time that might allow it to be named aloud. Different analysts have differing opinions on how much self-disclosure is appropriate. Meanwhile, a spiritual director simply holds it and waits and doesn't usually disclose if that would become an invitation to explore the transference relationship. But, in that holding, there is already a subtle invitation that gets thrown into the intersubjective pool between—a new openness, which can create empathy for the unspoken to be said by the directee. We need to be patient, intentional, and care-full, because what might have inhibited its expression could be shame, and it's not our job to expose it by excavating for this unspoken material.

3 Examine how the unspoken also might come out in an enactment—like a directee "forgetting" to come, or to pay. This can be dealt with straightforwardly as a "frame issue," keeping healthy boundaries, but keeping in mind that there might be a deeper meaning. Recognizing our countertransference as a clue to what might be going on is also a good way to not take things personally when the directee says or does something that we find hurtful. But as directors we stick to "where is Spirit in this, and what is Spirit trying to say to us both here?"

From Winnicott

From D. W. Winnicott (1965) we can maintain a "holding environment" that replicates the holding of the baby by the parent—a reliable, secure, and non-judgmental space for the directee to safely share their thoughts, and when things get sticky to neither abandon nor retaliate. We might also ask as Winnicott did, "Who holds the mother holding the baby?" Winnicott (1965), 37–55; Winnicott (1987), 17, 7 and in spiritual direction, just as in therapy, to seek out consultation or supervision when we find ourselves being unduly taxed or flummoxed by a particular directee's needs. That is to say, we can always be ready to refer for psychotherapy and not feel like we have to hold it all when it's beyond our own training, expertise, or role as spiritual director.

From Kohut

From Heinz Kohut, the founder of Self Psychology, we can not only find help in Kohut's emphasis on empathy, but a reminder that what Kohut meant by empathy was not a Rogerian definition of empathy as non-possessive warmth. Kohut (1982) viewed empathy as "vicarious introspection"—that is, trying as much as possible to understand from the patient's perspective what they are thinking, feeling, and experiencing, and then articulating it at the right time whether it is something "nice" or not. Kohut believed that empathy in itself was curative, perhaps in part because it is so rare. In a context of non-directive listening, I believe that to say "I am sensing x… I wonder if that resonates at all with you?" is an advanced form of mirroring, and not an intrusive interpretation. Especially because the client can always say "Nope, nothing to do with me." And then we just hold it, and don't press it. Sometimes it plants a seed, and sometimes we're just plain wrong!

Kohut's (1971, 1984) idea of "transmuting internalization" is also helpful here. Good active listening can go a long way toward helping the directee formulate their own provisional answers to questions, but at times there may be an impasse, or even a direct confrontation by the directee. In such an instance, we don't try to throw it back on them by analyzing their neuroticism! We acknowledge what we can—to the extent that it is true—and we express empathic concern. Often this is, for self psychologists, where the rubber really hits the road. We are disconfirming a negative response that the patient or directee is unconsciously expecting—maybe even unconsciously eliciting. And the experience of being heard rather than punished can shift something inside the patient—or directee. It's not a directee's job primarily to heal these old wounds, but sometimes the spiritual and the psychic do intersect in just such a way, and our response can be key to moving forward rather than hitting an irreversible impasse.

From Lacan

From Lacan, I also want to just pose the idea of the *sinthome*: "the idiosyncratic jouissance of a particular subject" (Verhaeghe and Declerq, 2002, p. 68). In my—admittedly limited—understanding of Lacanian theory, this means that each of us has a particular way of being neurotic that runs like a red thread through our relationship to: the Real—coming up against the external world, something like Freud's "necessity" which we can never fully grasp from our own subjective position; the symbolic—mainly how the Real is mediated to us through language and other symbolic forms; and the Imaginary—the meanings we make of what we experience within our subjectivity, and as we join together with others in creative meaning-making. This neuroticism shows itself in a characteristic symptom, but late in Lacan's theorizing he also called it the *sinthome* (Lacan, 2016 [2005]). That is, the characteristic ways in which we search for pleasure (*jouissance*) conditioned by everything that has happened to us previously in our lives. Perhaps also how we try to cope with jouissance when it becomes an excess of pleasure that we cannot stand any-more or comprehend. Related to spiritual direction, where does Lacan's jouissance touch on experiences of religious or spiritual ecstasy?

How do spiritual directors hold something as hot as that, especially when it raises a question of what is "genuine" spiritual experience, what is psychosis—or both? I will leave that for further reflection, but I don't think we can talk about *psyche* in either of its meanings—as soul or as mind—without leaving room for *ec-stasis*—moments of standing outside oneself either in mystical experience or psychotic break. Remember that in many schools of psychoanalysis including the Kleinian, relational, and Lacanian, we all are assumed to have a psychotic area or some aspect that is discontinuous with reality within our psyches. It's never easy to dis-entangle ecstasy from psychosis, and Lacan himself in his lecture on the *sinthome* interwove many examples of religion—as having an imaginary dimension—in a vertiginous dialogue with James Joyce's *Ulysses.* Perhaps this question is where the *sinthome* as irruption, as comma, as the "any-thing at all—but that," leads to a philosophical aporia. However, in such moments of in-breaking, spiritual directors are still left in their consulting rooms wondering quite practically what to do or say next. All we can do is hold the moment and trace the affect that follows. Perhaps at this juncture, all we can do is finally to fall back on the Ignatian idea of "discernment of spirits"—distinguishing good from evil—which St. Paul described as "love, joy, peace, patience, kindness, goodness, faithfulness, gentleness, self-control" (*Galatians*, 5:22–23, ESV). And could these not apply to other traditions beyond Christianity as well?

Conclusion

Finally, above all, I believe psychoanalysis and spiritual direction do share something, and it is not in theory, nor theology, nor listening technique, but it is a shared disposition.[9] That is, I believe, not seeking hard answers, but what the poet Rilke (1986 [1903]) described as "living the questions"—even "loving the questions":

> I would like to beg you dear Sir, as well as I can, to have patience with everything unresolved in your heart and to try to love the questions themselves as if they were locked rooms or books written in a very foreign language. Don't search for the answers, which could not be given to you now, because you would not be able to live them. And the point is to live everything. Live the questions now. Perhaps then, someday far in the future, you will gradually, without even noticing it, live your way into the answer.
>
> (p. 34)

Like St. Anselm, we embrace the mystery of G-d and ourselves as a multiplicity of *nescio quid*s ["I know not whats"][10] even as we discern certain cloudlike forms in the motion of the dance itself. These forms are the "truths" that emerge from either pastoral psychotherapy or spiritual direction—not *the* truth, but approximations and movements, pointing toward a horizon where understandings of selves and others shimmer ever more complexly.

Finally, both therapy/analysis and spiritual direction are processes of kenosis. We empty ourselves of all presumptions and presumptuousness, in order to enter a Trinitarian "third space" of metaphorical play and imagination. Empathy itself is kenosis. It is the self-emptying that relinquishes the need to "grasp" wisdom, or show off one's knowledge, inviting both caregiver and client into an intersubjective realm of exploration. In this intersubjective space, encapsulated and at times harmful fantasies and projections can be recognized and put in perspective, as mutual understanding can be tried on, practiced, and finally internalized as a habitus that is at once psychological, spiritual, and deeply ethical.

All of this requires a tolerance, even a deep reverence, in both types of practice, for silence, and for listening more than we speak. Analyst Sheldon Roth put this sensitivity beautifully into words when he wrote, "We want to behave as if excessive movement puts all of living nature into hiding, as it does at a woodland pond" (Roth, 2000, p. 441). Even with all the many revisions of psychoanalytic theory in the century since Freud, there is a primary quality of psychoanalytic therapy which is one of refraining and restraint. Freud's little motto, "When in doubt, don't," applies not only to unconsidered enactments, but to words as well. And the same goes for spiritual direction. Silence is not a stern "blank screen," but it is the ground out of which the work of psyche is encouraged to grow. This is the carer's discipline: to refrain from consciously adding anything extraneous, anything unconsidered, anything born of our own need. Enough will be added unconsciously—which is one of the best arguments for sitting still as much as possible. There is a stillness in both spiritual direction and analytically oriented practice that is not unlike Zen sitting. We wait, with complete attention.

We also wait with humility. The patient or directee is not an "It" to be acted on, but a "Thou" (Buber, 1970), a precious subject, as multiply and wonderfully constituted as we ourselves, and all living beings. As Martin

Buber cautioned, true I-Thou moments are fleeting; they cannot be grasped or manufactured. But practicing stillness, openness to the other, humility, and patient waiting may create the conditions of hospitality that make such moments more possible. This is the heart of the theological task: to be-with the one who comes to us for something—a deepening of spiritual formation, a desire to come closer to G-d/Spirit/the Sacred, a wrestling with vocation. They come to us not for us to be the expert on their life, their spirituality, but as a respectful guide like the poet Virgil was to the questing Dante—to that precious person's own winding journey into the *selva oscura*, the forest full of shadows. At the place of primordial silence, therapist and patient, director and directee, share a common humanity filled with both joy and suffering, and a common quest to understand the movement of Spirit in our lives. On such a journey, all are transformed.

Notes

1 E.g., psychoanalytic writings represented in the journal *Psychoanalytic Dialogues.*
2 SDI began as an ecumenical enterprise…envisioned and carried forward in 1989 at a conference of 90 spiritual directors at Mercy Center in Burlingame, California. Today it is known as Spiritual Directors International, with a membership that includes directors from over 50 nations representing multiple social, ethnic, and cultural traditions… Its journal *Presence: The Journal of Spiritual Directors International* has these aims: 'to facilitate professional conversation among spiritual directors and those engaged in the formation of spiritual directors' and 'to articulate the essential elements of our practice and training, to encourage accountability, and to develop clear ethical standards. (Wood, 2020, pp. 116–117) Originally centered in Christian spirituality, SDI has in the past decade expanded to encompass much wider inter-religious and spiritually fluid sources and practices.
3 These include a range of levels from one-time webinars (e.g., offered by SDI), certificate programs such as those offered at the Shalem Institute (Christian and multifaith), Stillpoint (Christian and multifaith), Columbia Theological Seminary (Protestant/Christian), the Yedidyah Center for Spiritual Direction (Jewish), Kol Dodi (Jewish), Upaya Zen Center (chaplaincy and end-of-life care programs) (Zen Buddhist); and graduate degree programs such as the Thich Nhat Hanh Program for Socially Engaged Buddhism (MDiv concentration) at Union Theological Seminary New York, as well as Master's programs offered at Loyola Marymount University (Roman Catholic/Ignatian and multifaith). There is a wealth of Roman Catholic/Ignatian training programs (listed on the Office of Ignatian Spirituality website), Buddhist retreat centers and programs (e.g., see the list on the Lion's Roar Buddhist directory website), and many, many more. (None of the above should be considered a formal endorsement.) The best place to begin is to find a spiritual director/companion through SDI to experience it for oneself, and then to explore local and online programs that best align with one's own spiritual tradition or pathway.
4 "Shalem is grounded in Christian contemplative spirituality and, at the same time, draws on the wisdom of many religious traditions." For more on the Shalem Institute, founded by Episcopal priest Tilden Edwards in 1973, see their website.
5 For more on intersubjectivity and using a relational psychoanalytic approach in spiritual and pastoral care, see Cooper-White (2007, 2011).

6 See also for a sample of recent articles and book reviews, SPT's *Journal of Pastoral Theology.*
7 Layton and others have been instrumental in founding Psychoanalysis for Social Responsibility, Section IX of Division 39 (the Society for Psychoanalysis and Psychoanalytic Psychology), of the American Psychological Association.
8 From a relational psychoanalytic perspective, see Bromberg (1998) and Davies (1998); from a relational pastoral theological perspective, see Cooper-White (2004, 2007, 2011).
9 This section is adapted and expanded from Cooper-White (2011): 242–243, 247.
10 In Anselm's *Monologion* 78, in S. N. Dean (Trans.) (1974), Saint Anselm: Basic Writings (Open Court), 142 as cited in Johnson (1994), 203.

References

Altman, R. (2009). *The analyst in the inner city: Race, class, and culture through a psychoanalytic lens*, 2nd ed. Routledge.

American Psychiatric Association. (2022). *Diagnostic and statistical manual of mental disorders* (5th ed., text rev.). American Psychiatric Association.

Belkin, M. and White, C. (2020). *Intersectionality and relational psychoanalysis: New perspectives on race, gender, and sexuality.* Routledge.

Benjamin, J. (2017). *Beyond doer and done to: Recognition theory, intersubjectivity, and the Third.* Routledge.

Bidwell, D. (2003). *Embedded psychologies and theologies: A foundation for critical theory in spiritual direction.* Unpublished PhD dissertation. Brite Divinity School.

Bidwell, D. (2004). Real/izing the sacred: Spiritual direction and social constructionism. *Journal of Pastoral Theology*, 14(1), 59–74.

Bregman, L. (2014). *The ecology of spirituality: Meanings, virtues, and practices in a post-religious age.* Baylor University Press.

Bromberg, P. (1998). *Standing in the spaces: Essays on clinical process, trauma, and dissociation.* Analytic Press.

Buber, M. (1970) *I and thou.* Kaufmann, W. (Trans.). Charles Scribner's.

Cataldo, L. (2008). Multiple selves, multiple Gods? Functional polytheism and the modern religious patient. *Pastoral Psychology* 57(1–2),45–58.

Cooper-White, P. (2004). *Shared wisdom: Use of the self in pastoral care and counseling.* Fortress.

Cooper-White, P. (2006). Thick theory: Psychology, theoretical models, and the formation of pastoral counselors. In Bidwell, D. and Marshall, J. (Eds.), *The formation of pastoral counselors: Challenges and opportunities* (pp. 47–68.) Haworth.

Cooper-White, P. (2007). *Many voices: Pastoral psychotherapy in relational and theological perspective.* Fortress.

Cooper-White, P. (2011). *Braided selves: Collected essays on multiplicity, God, and persons.* Cascade.

Cooper-White, P. (2012). Suffering. In Miller-McLemore, B. J. (Ed.), *The Wiley-Blackwell companion to practical theology* (pp. 23–31). Wiley Blackwell.

Cooper-White, P. (2018). *Old and dirty gods: Religion, antisemitism, and the origins of psychoanalysis.* Routledge.

Cooper-White, P. (2021). Paul Tillich's legacy in psychology and pastoral psychotherapy. In Bandy, T. G. (Ed.), *Why Tillich? Why now?* (pp. 191–206.) Mercer University Press.

Couture, P. (1991). *Blessed are the poor? Women's poverty, family policy, and practical theology.* Abingdon.

Cushman, P. (1995). *Constructing the self, constructing America: A cultural history of psychotherapy.* Addison-Wesley.

Davies, J.M. (1998). Multiple perspectives on multiplicity. *Psychoanalytic Dialogues*, 8, 195–206.

Ensign, J. (2023). *Depth calls to depth: Spiritual direction and Jungian psychology in dialogue.* Chiron.

Fanon, F. (2021). *Black skin, white masks.* Philcox, R. (Trans.) Penguin. (Orig. French publ. 1952.)

Fanon, F. (2004). *The wretched of the earth.* Philcox, R. (Trans.) Grove. (Orig. French publ. 1961.)

Fleming, D.L., SJ (2016). *Draw me into your friendship: The spiritual exercises – literal translation and contemporary reading*, (rev. ed.). Institute of Jesuit Sources.

Freud, S. (1961) The future of an illusion. In Strachey, J. (Ed. and Trans.) *The standard edition of the complete psychological works of Sigmund Freud*, 21 (pp. 1–56). Hogarth Press. (Orig. publ. 1927.)

Ganss, G. E., SJ (Ed.) (1991). *Ignatius of Loyola: Spiritual exercises and selected works.* Classics of Western spirituality. Paulist.

Gergen, K. (1999). *Invitation to social construction.* Sage.

Graham, L.K. (1992). *Care of persons, care of worlds: A psychosystems approach to pastoral care and counseling.* Abingdon.

Hart, T. (2005). Pastoral counseling or spiritual direction: What's the difference? *Presence: An International Journal of Spiritual Direction*, 11(2), 7–13.

Harter, M. (Ed.) (2005). *Hearts on fire: Praying with the Jesuits.* Loyola.

Ignatius of Loyola. (1999). *The spiritual exercises of St. Ignatius: or Manresa.* TAN Books. (Original work published 1522–1524.)

Jacoby, R. (1983). *The repression of psychoanalysis: Otto Fenichel and the political Freudians.* University of Chicago Press.

Johnson, E. (1994). *She who is: The mystery of God in feminist theological discourse.* Crossroad.

Jung, C.G. (2023). Jung on Ignatius of Loyola's Spiritual Exercises: Lectures delivered at ETH Zurich, Volume 7: 1939–1940. Philemon Foundation Series, 26. Liebscher, M. (Ed.), Stephens, C. (Trans.). Princeton University Press. (Orig. publ. as "The process of individuation: Exercitia spiritualia of St. Ignatius of Loyola: Notes on lectures given at the Eidgenössische Technische Hochschule, Zürich, June 1939–March 1940, *Modern Psychology*, 4.)

Kelsey, M. (1978). *Dreams: A way to listen to God.* Paulist.

Kohut, H. (1971). *The analysis of the self.* International Universities Press.

Kohut, H. (1984). *How does analysis cure?* Goldberg, A. and Stepansky, P. E. (Eds.). University of Chicago Press.

Kohut, H. (1982) Introspection, empathy, and the semi-circle of mental health. *International Journal of Psycho-analysis*, 63, 395–407.

Kuriloff, E. (2013). *Contemporary psychoanalysis and the legacy of the Third Reich.* Routledge.

Lacan, J. (2016). *The sinthome: The seminar of Jacques Lacan Book* XXII. Miller, J.-A. (Ed.), Price, A. R. (Trans.). Polity. (Orig. French publ. 2005.)

Layton, L. (2020). *Toward a social psychoanalysis: Culture, character, and normative unconscious processes.* Leavy-Sperounis, M. (Ed.). Routledge.
Layton, L., Hollander, N.C. and Gutwill, S. (Eds.). (2006). *Psychoanalysis, class and politics: Encounters in the clinical setting.* Routledge.
Lion's Roar Buddhist Directory. Website at https://directory.lionsroar.com/. Accessed June 21, 2026.
Noth, I. and Morgenthaler, C. (2014). The friendship between Sigmund Freud and Oskar Pfister. *Pastoral Psychology*, 63, 81–90.
Ogden, T. (2004). The analytic third: Implications for psychoanalytic theory and technique. *Psychoanalytic Quarterly*, 73(1), 167–195.
Oliver, M. (1990). *House of Light.* Beacon Press.
Office of Ignatian Spirituality. Website at https://www.jesuitseastois.org/. Accessed June 19, 2026.
Pfister, O. (1993). The illusion of a future: A friendly disagreement with Prof. Sigmund Freud. Roazen, P. (Ed.) Abrams, S. and Taylor, T. (Trans.) *International Journal of Psycho-Analysis*, 74, 557–579. (Orig. German publ. 1928.)
Ramsay, N. (2018). *Pastoral theology and care: Critical trajectories in theory and practice.* Wiley-Blackwell.
Reik, T. (1948). *Listening with the third ear: The inner experience of the psychoanalyst.* Farrar, Straus.
Rilke, R. M. (1986). *Letters to a young poet.* Mitchell, S. (Trans.). Vintage. (Orig. publ. 1903.)
Roth, S. (2000). *Psychotherapy: The art of wooing nature.* Jason Aronson. (Orig. publ. 1987.)
Sanford, J. A. (1989). *Dreams: God's forgotten language*, (rev. ed.). HarperOne.
SDI (n.d.) *Spiritual Directors International.* Website at https://www.sdicompanions.org/. Accessed June 17, 2026.
Shalem Institute for Spiritual Formation. Website at https://shalem.org/. Accessed June 19, 2026.
SPT (n.d.) *Society for pastoral theology.* Website at https://www.societyforpastoraltheology.org. Retrieved June 17, 2026.
Tillich, P. (1957). *Dynamics of faith.* Harper and Row.
Tillich, P. (1959). The theology of pastoral care. *Pastoral Psychology*, 10(7), 21–26.
Verhaeghe, P. and Declarcq, F. (2002). Lacan's goal of analysis: Le sinthome or the feminine way. In Thurston, L. (Ed.), *Re-inventing the symptom: Essays on the final Lacan*. Other Press.
Winnicott, C.W. (1987). *Babies and their mothers.* Addison-Wesley.
Winnicott, D. W. (1965). *The maturational processes and the facilitating environment: Studies in the theory of emotional development.* Karnac.
Wood, N. S. (2020). Pastoral counseling and spiritual direction: Pastoral theology's stepchildren? In Stjerna, K. and Schramm, B., (Eds.) *Spirituality: Toward a 21st century Lutheran understanding* (pp. 109–120.) Augsburg Fortress.
Yalom, I. (1989). *Love's executioner and other tales of psychotherapy.* Basic Books.

Chapter 4

Divine Paradox

The Centrality of Metaphor in the Work of Spiritual Direction

Alden B. Flanders

For Otto Schoen-Rene

We say that in any one-on-one spiritual direction session there are three present: the directee, the director, and God. Some of us place a third chair facing the chairs of the director and the directee. What is the status of that chair? Is it for God to sit in? Well, of course not. God, the ultimate, as understood by many traditions, certainly by the three Abrahamic faiths, is beyond human knowledge and understanding. God is infinite and unknowable, unbounded by anything in creation, much less a chair. Any director or directee who thinks God literally sits in that chair has problems. So, no, God doesn't sit in that chair. But if that is true, why bother? "Here, let me put out this third chair that God isn't sitting in." The reality is that we put the chair there to make concrete the spiritual presence of God.

What does that mean, how does it work, making concrete the presence of God, or of any intangible entity, reality, being? The chair, by itself, asserts nothing, it is just a chair. The assertion that the chair is God's is a function of language, of a particular use of language. It is not verifiable, scientific language; it is imaginative language that is shared within a community—in the present context, the community of the spiritual director and the person who is looking to deepen their spiritual life, whom we will call the directee. This imaginative language takes on a particular pattern and has an ancient heritage; it is the language of metaphor.

As Janet Martin Soskice (1985, p. 17) says in her book, *Metaphor and Religious Language*:

> He who points to the daffodils in the garden and says that they are metaphors for rebirth speaks carelessly and indeed metaphorically. Daffodils are not in themselves and could not be metaphors, for they are not linguistic at all. [One] can reasonably say that the daffodil is a symbol of rebirth or that it provides an analogy for rebirth, since neither the category of symbol nor that of analogy is strictly linguistic. However, although we can construct a metaphor in which we speak of daffodils in order to describe rebirth, the daffodils themselves are not metaphors.

DOI: 10.4324/9781003742852-4

In the same way, whoever points to the third chair in the spiritual direction room can say that it is a symbol; but, in exploring the role of metaphor in spiritual direction, we are exploring the uses of language. Therefore, the chair is an artifact about which we speak in a metaphorical way.

The use of metaphorical language in regard to that third chair is a way of affirming that God is present, even at the very moment we know that God is not present in any sense we can describe in language. This is the central paradox of metaphor, that it tells us the truth of something by making a statement about that something that is demonstrably false, or fictive. If I tell my directee that God is sitting in that third chair, I am not telling a literal truth; just as Romeo does not tell the truth when he says Juliet is the sun. But I am telling a spiritual truth: our metaphorical language about the chair calls us into relationship with God. At the same time, as we respond to the mystery of the presence of God, that same language reaches down and opens for us the door to our inner life.

The Nature of Spiritual Direction

So, what is spiritual direction? The many directors conducting the practice may have a wide range of answers to this question, but from my own experience as a directee and a director, I would describe spiritual direction as a discipline of intense listening, focused understanding, and deepening questioning. Spiritual direction is a work that demands intense humility, a terrible withholding of judgment, a probing honesty, and a transforming compassion. It demands of us that we should have, not certainty, not answers to all the questions, but a groundedness, a relationship with the ultimate, with God, that frees us from the need to be right, to be in control. It is here that we come up against the contradiction in the use of the word "direction" for the work that we do. In spiritual direction we do not direct—or perhaps I should say, we do not direct very often; but when we direct it is with the deepest compassionate authority, which is the authority, not of our ego, or of tenure, but of experience tempered by humility grounded in our relationship with God.

Unlike the counseling offered by a pastor to a parishioner, spiritual direction occurs in a regular rhythm, often monthly, and there is normally no other contact between director and directee in between sessions. Again, unlike pastoral counseling, direction is not focused on solving problems in a person's life, but on the directee's relationship with God. The directee sets the agenda; their problems will come up in the conversation, but the focus of the work is not the solution of the problems, but how those problems offer insight into the working of God in a person's life. And so, another of the skills demanded of a spiritual director is patience. It may take months or years for the relationship with God to deepen, for issues to gel, for the directee's fundamental images to come forward and clarify, for the skills and understanding of the directee to develop.

Our work as spiritual directors demands a discipline that knows the lore and the heritage of spiritual practice through different traditions and different ages. And spiritual direction asks us to be able to recognize the stories and images that give a directee access to their inner life so that we can assist our directees in the adventure of discovery, both of their inner world and of the reality of God, as that knowledge unfolds over time. It is this part of the spiritual director's work, the recognition and bringing to bear of the images that define and give access to the inner person, that is the focus of this chapter, for these images are metaphors and the understanding of them and the sharing of that understanding between directee and director is at the heart of our work.

Metaphor: Our Only Language for God

I suspect that we all have some intuitive sense that metaphor is important in spiritual practice and in our work of spiritual direction. If nothing else we know that metaphor allows us to name the unnameable, to begin to give some shape and understanding to the nature and content of our inner lives. And of course, the place where the darkness of our inner lives and the mystery of our outer lives meet, is in God, the ultimate.

David Tracy, Professor of Catholic Studies, Theology, and the Philosophy of Religions at the University of Chicago Divinity School, specializes in the study of religion and religious traditions in a multicultural world. He approaches this study by looking at the ways language shapes our knowledge of God and the ways we talk about God. In an essay in Sheldon Sacks's collection, *On Metaphor* (1979), Tracy says, "All major religions are grounded in certain root metaphors" (Tracy, 1979, p. 89). He affirms that all the great religious traditions use metaphor to speak of the realities that are beyond our grasp and our understanding. He develops the concept of root metaphors—the fundamental, defining metaphors of the great religious traditions that express and shape each religion's sense of ultimacy. Over the centuries these metaphors have been explored, their ramifications teased out, changed, developed. These root metaphors are the basis on which theology and spiritual practice are built, defining belief and shaping the experience of the presence of God.

In his book, *Blessed Rage for Order*, Tracy (1975) develops his phenomenological study of theology and religious language by reference to an understanding of the human situation as a reality that is limited. It is limited by our finite nature, limited by the reality of our death. As human beings we find ourselves in what he calls this "limit-situation" and our conceptual, analytical ways of understanding the human condition share the limits of our finite nature. Tracy says that it is only "symbolic" language that can express the unspeakable nature of what it means to confront the anxiety of this "limit-situation." Tracy is not always clear in his use of the categories of metaphorical and symbolic language. Thus, when he speaks of "symbolic language," I interpret that he wants to include non-linguistic symbols as well as metaphor in his presentation. The relevance of his thought to the present work is, I believe, clear. Tracy draws on fundamental existential ideas to build his presentation of our condition.

Anxiety is literally, as Heidegger reminds us, a fear of No-thing…

> More positively stated, anxiety is a fear disclosive of our often forgotten but never totally absent consciousness of our own radical contingency. … [W]e find ourselves—as the metaphors of the existentialists and the mystics alike remind us—poised over an abyss, a chasm, whose exact nature we do not know but whose experiential reality we cannot deny.
>
> (Tracy, 1975, p. 107)

But this perilous vista leads to something more.

> At a certain point the language of conceptual analysis begins to falter. Instead, the human spirit begins to search for metaphors expressive of the experience (abyss, chasm, limit) and for narratives capable of expanding and structuring these metaphors (parables, myths, poems). Such metaphors, images, symbols, and myths seem linguistically necessary to express that literally unspoken, and perhaps unspeakable, final dimension to the end of our lives. In a word, the language initially most appropriate for expressing that experience is symbolic as distinct from strictly conceptual. Such language, as symbolic, involves a double intentionality which expresses both a literal meaning (for example, an actual physical abyss) and a non-literal meaning which otherwise remains unsaid and unspoken.
>
> …All authentic limit-language seems to be initially and irretrievably a symbolic and metaphorical one. Insofar as the hidden dimension of an ultimate limit is not merely hidden but not even expressible in the language of the everyday … that language retains the linguistic structure of metaphor and symbol. … even *explicitly* religious language (e.g., the language of the scriptures or of the Christian mystics) is intrinsically symbolic and metaphorical limit-language.
>
> (Tracy, 1975, pp. 107–108)

Tracy thus makes the movement to metaphor fundamental to the human condition—a condition inexorably tied to a pointing toward what cannot be expressed yet toward which we strive.

Another author who explores the use of metaphors in the building of a theology is Sallie McFague. As a Protestant and feminist theologian, in her book *Metaphorical Theology: Models of God in Religious Language* (1982) she looks to free religious language and tradition from the dominance of patriarchal imagery. In order to do this, she builds a theology, not on doctrines or dogmas, but on metaphor. Her focus is on the parables of Jesus as extended metaphors that do not dictate a particular interpretation or creed, but, like all metaphors, allow for a broad range of interpretation. She then looks at Jesus himself as a parable, as a metaphor.

Rather than see traditional metaphors by which God is identified as essential and unchangeable, McFague (1982) reminds us that metaphor is both true and false, expresses a truth by making a false statement, and therefore all metaphors for God hold some truth, but are also limited in their application. "One significant difference between symbolic and metaphorical statements is that the latter always contain the whisper, 'it is *and it is not*'" (p. 9).

> If metaphor is the way by which we understand as well as enlarge our world and change it—that is, if the only way we have of dealing with the unfamiliar and new is in terms of the familiar and the old, thinking of "this" as "that" although we know the new thing is both like *and* unlike the old—if all this is the case, then it is no surprise that Jesus taught in parables or that many see him as a parable of God. For he introduced a new, strange way of being in the world, a way that could be grasped only through the indirection of stories of familiar life which both "were and were not" the kingdom.
>
> (McFague, 1982, p. 18)

McFague's purpose in building a theology based on metaphor, is to urge that no metaphor is the only, the defining way to talk about God, and that we need to use a richer palette of metaphors to describe a God who cannot be trapped in purely masculine imagery. Basing her theology on the parables, and on the life of Jesus himself, allows her to build diverse metaphorical imagery in a series of characteristics of those parables, and of Jesus' ministry itself.

Since Jesus' metaphorical stories and parables use as their images everyday relationships among people, McFague (1982) can define her metaphorical theology as personal and relational, and to do so more broadly than the tradition has usually done. In order to build her metaphorical theology, McFague defines layers of metaphorical language and the ways that language functions in allowing clear and logically lucid conceptual statements. The first layer of metaphorical language is the metaphor itself, where it is asserted that A is B: Jesus is the shepherd. The second order is the root metaphor, model, or "...a dominant metaphor, a metaphor with staying power" (p. 23). This root metaphor, or model, defines and shapes the understanding, using the idea of root metaphor in the same sense as David Tracy. "God is father" is such a model, where fatherhood is seen as a defining image for God. Its power, of course, is part of the problem; thus, McFague wants to focus on a range of root metaphors.

Beyond this root metaphor or model, says McFague (1982), the metaphor is generalized into a level of abstraction as a concept and theory.

> Concepts and theories arise from metaphors and models, they are an attempt to generalize at the level of abstraction concerning competing and, at times, contradictory metaphors and models. By "concept" we mean an abstract notion; by "theory" we mean a speculative, systematic statement of relationships underlying certain phenomena. A concept is an idea or thought; a theory organizes ideas into an explanatory structure. Concepts, unlike metaphors, do not create new meaning, but rely on conventional, accepted meanings. Theories, unlike models, do not systematize one area in terms of another, but organize concepts into a whole.
>
> (pp. 25–26)

Both Tracy and McFague recognize the centrality of metaphor in understanding religious language in any modern attempt to make sense of the assertions of theology. Tracy's work uses metaphor to help Christians be secure in their beliefs while in dialog with their neighbors of other faiths or of no faith. McFague's work uses an understanding of metaphor to expand the repertoire of images that can move Christians beyond the limits of patriarchy. In the present work, I am exploring metaphor not only as the way we can speak about God, but as the way we can speak about our experience of God in the context of spiritual direction. And thus, it makes sense to look in some depth at how one of the classical spiritual directors uses metaphor.

John of the Cross: Metaphors that Negate Images

We will begin to see the role of metaphor in the work of spiritual direction if we look at the work of John of the Cross (1529–1591), friend, advisor, and spiritual director of Teresa of Avila (1515–1582) and her nuns. He was one of the great mystics, great spiritual directors, and one of the great psychologists of the spiritual life. At the heart of his work are two fundamental beliefs: the first is that God is unknowable, the second is the metaphorical statement that God is love. John says, in his commentary to *The Living Flame of Love* (1585–1591):

> God transcends the intellect and is incomprehensible and inaccessible to it. Hence, when the intellect is understanding, it is not approaching God, but withdrawing from him. It must withdraw from itself and from its knowledge, so as to journey to God in faith, by believing and not understanding. It reaches God more by not understanding than by understanding.
>
> (Saint John of the Cross, 1991, p. 692)

John is leery of the use of the imagination in the spiritual life. He acknowledges that it may be necessary for those beginning their journey to God to use imagination, to use images in meditation; but very quickly the directee must give up the use of imagination and images. The renunciation of images is one of the conditions that allows the directee to enter the dark night of purgation, which is dark precisely because we put aside all our images of God, all our assumptions about God, all that we project onto God. The dark night prepares the soul for betrothal and union with God. And this state is image-free because it is God who reaches into the soul of the directee and leads it on; it is not the effort of the directee, or of the director. And, in order to speak about this imageless state, John piles metaphor upon metaphor, "dark night," "ascent," "betrothal," "marriage," "union," all building upon the fundamental metaphor that says that "God is Love."

Why did John of the Cross feel that it was acceptable to use these metaphors to talk about the dangers of images? Or was he simply a literalist about all these metaphors of God's love? Perhaps, but anyone who so radically espouses the apophatic stance of the unknowability of God would have trouble being a literalist of that sort. Did John recognize that a metaphor is not an image, at least in the sense that he uses the word? A metaphor is not a static assertion claiming the truth or reality of something. As McFague (1982) points out, metaphor exists in a state of tension, claiming an identity between two things that are not identical. Shakespeare (1564–1616)—John of the Cross's contemporary—has Romeo assert that "It is the East and Juliet is the sun" (*Romeo and Juliet*, 1597/2016, 2.2.3). Yet, Juliet is not the sun; Juliet is not a huge ball of flaming gases. To assert that Juliet is the sun in any literal sense is nonsense. But when Romeo says that Juliet is the sun, he tells us a great deal about his own inner life and about the qualities of the sun that he associates with Juliet: warmth, life, nurture. And is it possible that in the mind of Shakespeare, consciously or unconsciously, the image of Juliet as the rising sun is associated with resurrection, the rising of the son of God and the giving of new life?

Almost the whole of the life and work of John of the Cross, in prose and poetry, and in his work with St. Teresa and her nuns, is an exploration of the ramifications of the metaphor, "God is love." His best-known work—by its title if not by its content—*The Dark Night* (of the Soul) (1578/1579; commentary 1584–1585) is not a guide about what to do when life is difficult, it is a challenge to choose the apophatic way, the *via negativa*, a life of contemplation and self-denial. John sees the spiritual life as beginning with a dark night of deprivation and purgation so that the directee may come through the darkness of the unknowable to the breaking in of the light wholly transformed by the love of God. In the tradition of earlier Christian mysticism, John's later works take the biblical *Song of Songs*. Using this love poetry as an extended metaphor, he explores the metaphor of love, going deeper and deeper, understanding that the bride in the *Song* is the soul, the bridegroom is Christ, and the work of the directee is to prepare for the union with God as the bride prepares for the marriage. It's easy to snigger at the sexuality in John's work, as though, as a monastic, he didn't understand the eroticism of what he was saying. But he was in a long tradition of Christian spirituality that uses the *Song of Songs* as a metaphor for the union of the soul with God. In spite of the erotic quality of some of his verses and his prose, it's clear that he knew exactly what he was saying. He was following the metaphor of the love of God as far as it could go in human terms.

I suspect that John of the Cross used metaphor because he knew that this wild and shifting use of falsehood was the only way to help his directees avoid the traps of the intellect and to live deeply into the practices that would unite them with God, helping them to experience the truth and the love of God. Because metaphor claims an identity between two clearly unrelated things, its truth lies in the gut, the intuition, the heart rather than in the orderly organization of the intellect. It is an understanding of a vastly different order from the rational intellectual disciplines.

The tension between the untruth that the metaphor tells and the truth it implies drives inquiry, a search that seeks to satisfy intellectual curiosity; but, even more, a search that drives us inward to seek a resolution of the tension in self-knowledge and serenity.

Metaphor and the Shaping of Lives

What is there about metaphor that shapes lives? Isn't metaphor simply a rhetorical trick, a way to play with words? I. A. Richards (2001 [1936]), in a series of lectures at Bryn Mawr in 1936, revolutionized and revitalized the field of metaphor studies. Because of Richards's work, metaphor has become one of the central concerns in linguistic studies and the philosophy of language. Richards's contention was that metaphor is more than a trick of rhetoric, it is the great paradoxical fountain of creativity, of building new cognitive worlds. And it does this because it forces an identity between things in radically different domains. It forces a juxtaposition that shocks us out of our assumed and accepted ways of looking at the world and creates new possibilities. As James Geary (2011) says in his popular and accessible overview of recent metaphor scholarship, *I is an Other*, a metaphor tells us what a thing is by telling us what it is not. Or as Italian scholar and psychoanalyst, Gemma Corradi Fiumara (1995, p. 11), whose work I will discuss in greater depth later on, says, "The paradox of a metaphor is that it seems to affirm an identity while also somehow denying it."

Metaphor takes belief out of the realm of scientific proof and returns it to a place of mystery and awe. Metaphor unites disparate worlds. In metaphor we equate two unlike, dissimilar things. One of those things we know well, the other we do not know, or we want to know better. And we declare that these two dissimilar things are identical: Juliet is the sun; America is a melting pot; my kid's room is a disaster area; the brain is a computer; heart of gold; hit the sack; bite the bullet; bent out of shape; hit the nail on the head. Or the foundational metaphor of that great spiritual director, Dante Alighieri:

> Midway this way of life we're bound upon
> I woke to find myself in a dark wood,
> Where the right road was wholly lost and gone.
> (Dante Alighieri, 1949 [1320], Sayers Translation, I:1–3)

But each individual metaphor is part of a larger process, each metaphor is an example of the fundamental way we explore reality and build our worlds of thought and dreams. I. A. Richards (2001 [1936]) says that metaphor is not just a form of words, but that metaphoric thinking is the way we make sense of the world and the way we relate to each other. Metaphoric process is the root of all language, it is the means of all exploration and the path to discovery, and not only poetic or religious discovery, but scientific as well. Metaphor allows us to gain some understanding of things that we do not yet understand, it allows us to give a name and shape to the unknown and the unknowable.

Richards (2001 [1936]) asserts that the nature of the mind and the nature of metaphor are yoked, so that the metaphoric process, which claims the identity of unlike things, claims the interest and attention of the mind, whose very nature is to connect unlike things:

> Let us consider more closely what happens in the mind when we put together—in a sudden and striking fashion—two things belonging to very different orders of experience [as in the two elements of a metaphor]. The most important happenings... are the mind's efforts to connect them. The mind is a connecting organ, it works only by connecting and it can connect any two things in an indefinitely large number of different ways. Which of these it chooses is settled by reference to some larger whole or aim.... The reader [or, as in spiritual direction, listener]... will try out various connections and this experimentation... is the movement which gives meaning to all fluid language.
> (p. 84)

Richards then goes on to point out that metaphors are made up of words, and it is the form of these words that brings together the things that are not in themselves combinable:

> Words are the meeting points at which regions of experience which can never combine in sensation or intuition, come together. They are the occasions and means of that growth which is the mind's endless endeavour to order itself. That is why we have language... It is the instrument of all our distinctively human development.
> (p. 88)

By demanding that we use our imagination and our intuition, metaphor takes us out of our heads and into the deep places of the heart and the spirit. And so I say that metaphor is the root and the route of the inner life—it opens the door to our deepest, inchoate thoughts and feelings. Metaphor gives us access to our own creative lives, to that rich broth that nourishes our truest humanity.

We can, of course, deny the power of metaphor in our lives; this is called literalism, and literalism makes us rigid black and white thinkers. Fiumara (1995, p. 135) says, "Literalism deprives us of our expressive resources. We don't need to translate from our inner world to sharable language. We lose the ability to recognize our inner world." And isn't that one important, centrally important, aspect of our work as directors; to encourage, and to listen as our directees struggle to translate from their inner worlds into the sharable language of our time together? I don't think I'm wrong when I say that an awareness of and sensitivity to metaphor is one of the most important tools in a spiritual director's repertoire.

Fiumara takes us deeper into the power of metaphor to shape the inner life. She is a psychoanalyst and a philosopher of language. She focuses on the dynamics of language in the interaction of the speaker who wants to be understood, and the listener who wants to understand. Her work helps us to see how metaphor gives the directee access to their inner life; how it binds director and directee together, and helps the directee/director team to make exciting discoveries in the inner world. Her book *The Metaphoric Process* (1995) explores the role of metaphor in this dynamic of listener and speaker, of seeker and helper. It is a great resource for those of us who do spiritual direction; for, though we are not therapists or analysts, we are listeners who are engaged with the inner lives of those to whom we offer spiritual companionship.

In order to develop her ideas about dialog, Fiumara (1995, p. 27) begins with her assumptions about metaphor and the inner life: "In order to try to describe the unknown we must resort to concepts that we know—that is the basic effect of metaphor: an unusual juxtaposition of the familiar and the unfamiliar." In other words, to name and describe what we do not know, or cannot describe, we use language that describes what we do know. Juliet, whom Romeo is only beginning to know, is equated with the sun, which he does know, at least in its impact on him. Other metaphors show up regularly in spiritual direction for Christians: God is love; Jesus is the good shepherd; my life is a journey; in the middle of my life, I found myself in a dark wood. Metaphor thus becomes the means by which we can use the things we know to identify the unknown reality of our inner self. Fiumara (1995, p. 55) says, speaking not only as a philosopher, but as someone engaged in dialog with her patients for the discovery of their inner lives, "The use of metaphoric language appears to be interwoven with the actual development of our inner lives.".

A directee struggles to explore and discover the metaphors that define the shape of their inner landscape and the characters in their inner drama. As they struggle to express that landscape and the characters that inhabit it, the conversation between director and directee becomes affirmation for the searcher and helps to bring the images into focus. Fiumara (1995, p. 119) says, "Metaphor is an indivisible process of both construction and construal." Thus the directee constructs the metaphors that connect the inchoate inner life with the known realities of the outer life. At the same time the director, or in Fiumara's case, the analyst, construes those metaphors and hears and accepts them, affirming the tentative images of the directee and coming up with a shared idea of the spiritual identity of the directee.

For Fiumara the process of growth and maturity, the inner journey, depends on the presence of a listener attuned to that inner work and sensitive to the metaphors that are constructed in the process. Fiumara writes:

> An appropriate response [by the listener] to non-literal [that is, metaphoric] dialog convinces the individual that the inner world can be thought about and articulated. If metaphors are not listened to and joined in with, no consensual thinking could properly develop... It is only through the creative listening of others that our expressions of the experiences we live through but cannot yet think of can be linked with mature levels of articulation.
>
> (Fiumara, 1995, p. 139)

Part of this work of dialog is involved with letting the metaphors guide us and our directees. Thus, not every metaphor holds the same value. According to Fiumara (1995, p. 126), "Basic metaphors can be identified which guide one's life journey by the constant process of shaping a diachronic, enduring structure of the self." In other words, the inner self is shaped by the application and interpretation of the root metaphors—as in McFague's models—that arise from and apply to many times across the range of our life's experiences. Some of these are metaphors that we generate ourselves, but many are provided by the culture, and taken in, and made our own. These may come from the arts and popular culture, from science, from philosophy, and from other places. One of the challenges of the spiritual life, one of our challenges as directors, is to bring together the metaphors that arise from our directees' own experiences, the ones that speak to them from the culture around them, and the metaphors that come from our various religious traditions. Part of our work is to help our directees see that metaphor invites—demands—flexibility and playfulness. We need to try to gently wean them off any residual literalism that they hold on to for security.

The work of our basic metaphors, root metaphors, is to guide us along the path and into greater self-knowledge. In Fiumara's words:

> To make explicit the ramifications of our dominant metaphors is to engage in a practice that brings us inexorably closer to our inner life. This enhances the shifts and dynamics of our relationships with our culture. This grounds our work in an historic community of living creatures.
>
> (Fiumara, 1995, p. 85)

She calls metaphors "inchoate explanatory devices" (p. 12), where the boundary between the poetic and the heuristic is unclear, and points to the heuristic use of metaphor as an agent of discovery. These basic metaphors that guide our lives are in part poetry, but they are also heuristics that guide and shape our inner lives; and in shaping our inner lives they shape our outer lives, as well as our moral and ethical lives.

Our work as spiritual directors has a great deal to do with what Fiumara (1995, p. 85) calls "the ramifications of our dominant metaphors." In explaining his understanding of the root metaphors of a tradition, Catholic theologian David Tracy (1979, p. 89) argues, "In a particular religion root metaphors form a cluster or network in which certain sustained metaphors both organize subsidiary metaphors and diffuse new ones." Our work is to help our directees discover the shape that these clusters of root metaphors take in their own inner lives, and how these clusters guide them on their journey of faith and spiritual practice. The metaphors around kingship can take us in one direction, those concerned with fatherhood in another, and motherhood, as McFague (1982) points out, in another.

Belief: Dogma, Doctrine, and Metaphor

Root metaphors play multiple roles in the life of the faith community and of believers. Over the millennia of the Christian Era, certain root metaphors have been determined by the authority structures of the various faith communities, denominations, or churches as being essential to Christian identity and belief. This is not the place to trace a history of creeds, ecumenical councils, papal bulls, and the various protestant statements of belief, both mainline and evangelical. It is enough to say that almost all Christian bodies have ways of defining their central and non-negotiable beliefs and of making clear that commitment to that community of faith involves a public statement of acceptance and belief.

Doctrines and dogmas are authoritative statements of what the members of a faith community are expected to affirm or believe. The form of these statements of belief, such as the creeds, is usually, "I believe in A, B, and C." How often do pastors hear parishioners say, with some asperity, "Why do we have to say the creeds? I don't believe that stuff," or "I just don't say the parts of the creed that I don't believe." Doctrines and dogmas are presented as baseline non-negotiables, meaning that you can't be a member if you can't say the creed, or whatever affirmation of faith is central for that particular community.

But these statements of faith are not declarations of affirmation that the terms of the statement are scientifically, literally true. These statements of faith are listings of the root metaphors of that community of faith, usually in a narrative form, and metaphors, as we have said, are both true and not true; they are false statements that tell a truth. Therefore, whatever the requirements of the authority structures of a community of faith, as a spiritual director, my primary interest is in the role a metaphor plays in the life of faith of my directee.

Consider the Apostles' Creed. It presents a series of doctrinal assertions in the form of statements of belief. But those statements of belief either are themselves metaphoric, or derive from fundamental root metaphors of Christianity:

> I believe in God, the Father almighty,
> creator of heaven and earth;
> I believe in Jesus Christ, his only Son, our Lord.
> He was conceived by the power of the Holy Spirit
> and born of the Virgin Mary.
> He suffered under Pontius Pilate,
> was crucified, died, and was buried.
> He descended to the dead.
> On the third day he rose again.
> He ascended into heaven,
> and is seated at the right hand of the Father.
> He will come again to judge the living and the dead.
> I believe in the Holy Spirit,
> the holy catholic Church,
> the communion of saints,
> the forgiveness of sins
> the resurrection of the body,
> and the life everlasting. Amen.
> (From the *Book of Common Prayer* of the Episcopal Church in the United States, 1979)

Consider the metaphors in the Apostles' Creed:

- God is **God**, God is **Father**, God is **almighty**, God is **creator**, of **heaven.**
- Jesus is the **Son** of God, the **only** son of God, is our **Lord.**
- Jesus was conceived by the **Holy Spirit** and given birth by the **Virgin Mary.**
- Jesus **suffered** and was **crucified, died**, and was **buried.** (As part of a mythic narrative these elements are also metaphoric.)
- Jesus **descended to the dead**; on the third day he **rose** and **ascended into heaven,** where he sits at **the right hand of God.**
- Jesus is **judge** and will **come again.**
- The power of God is the **Holy Spirit** (wind, or breath) who empowers the **catholic Church** and the **communion of saints,** enables the **forgiveness of sins,** the **resurrection of the body**, and the life everlasting.
- And, of course, embedded in the creed, in its content and its form, is the **Doctrine of the Trinity.**

Apart from its doctrinal or dogmatic significance, each of these metaphors will have resonances in the faith and inner life of our directees. As noted above, the resonances and ramifications of God as father are the subject of Sallie McFague's *Metaphorical Theology* (1982) and have been a matter of active theological debate in churches for the last half century and more. But for our directees, the metaphor of God as father will in addition carry associations with their own personal fathers, father figures, clergy who may carry the title Father, and perhaps: associations with Darth Vader and Luke Skywalker; King Charles and his two boys; Carson Drew and Nancy; Atticus Finch and Scout; or even Noah Cross and Evelyn Mulwray from Polanski's *Chinatown* (1974).

I believe that part of our work as spiritual directors is to help our directees clarify the difference between the use of metaphors by church authorities and the use of metaphors in our awareness of our inner life and its growth. And in order to do this we have to help them understand the nature and the power of metaphor, and its use in our spiritual lives. Some of our directees will be sophisticated and aware of the role of metaphor; but many more will, I suspect, have a surface awareness of metaphor but not be able to distinguish the demands of authority from the uses of the imagination in the development of the inner life. And many of these directees, again superficially aware of metaphor, will still be struggling with the implications of literalness in the recitation of the creeds. When asked whether they believe in God, the Incarnation, the Virgin Birth, or the Trinity, they will be trapped in the anxiety of having to give a yes or no answer. Part of our work with directees is to help them, as they honestly explore their inner lives, to know that the recitation of the creed is a symbolic act—the Greek word for the creeds is, in fact, σύμβολον [*symbolum*]. As a symbolic act, the recitation of the creeds is an act of unity and solidarity with the community of faith and an affirmation of the historical continuity of the scriptural narrative and its power in the lives of Christians.

Some of our directees will be more anxious about and more wedded to a literal understanding of the creeds than others. We will need to be gentle as they take the journey from the literal to the metaphoric. And our goal is not to destroy their literal belief, but to help them make the discovery that God does not want them to be anxious, but to find the place of faith in their hearts where they can see the figurative nature of the myth as a gift of God embedded in the very language that is one of the fundamental metaphors for Jesus Christ: The Word.

Think for a moment about what is probably the most basic and the most misunderstood metaphor of all: God. When I was teaching religion as an academic subject to high school students, one of our texts was Paul Tillich's *Dynamics of Faith* (1957). Buried in Tillich's difficult prose, he says, "God is a symbol of God" (Tillich, 1957, p. 46). This drove my kids nuts. Tillich was filled with incomprehensible language and ideas, but this idea of God as a symbol of God was beyond difficult. This was learnéd nonsense and they felt like someone—Tillich, or the teacher, or the universe—someone was having them on and shaming them. For my students, Tillich's language about God was nonsense, but Fiumara (1995) says that metaphor makes sense of nonsense. And isn't that what St. Paul is saying in First Corinthians (*I Corinthians* 1:25, NTFE) "For God's foolishness is wiser than human wisdom, and God's weakness is stronger than human strength"?

The word "God," is a metaphor for the unknowable mystery to which we give the label, God. That first word "God," helps us know the ultimate mystery that is the second word God, by doing what metaphors do. It receives all of our cultural projections and assumptions about the divine, the ultimate—call it what you will. It is this first "God" who has been traditionally addressed as male, who is the old man in the sky whom people don't believe in; but this first word "God" helps us because it relates the unknowable God to the things we do know, even if with time and changing cultural norms and the advance of science, we find much of the accretion around that first "God" unacceptable, or unbelievable. God may not be male, may not be an old man, may not be angry, may not live in a heavenly city with streets paved with gold. Yet certain metaphors associated with the metaphor "God" have lasted and given us a sense of the nature of the unknowable God behind "God": God is love, is justice, is healer; God calls us into mature human community. These are root metaphors that outlast the metaphors that fed other people at other times, root metaphors that can still sustain us. But these are the revelations by which the ultimate mystery still hides itself. It is only by looking at our human experience that we are given a hint—a hint followed by guesses—of the God beyond God. Imagine the irony that by being literalists and believing only in the first expression of God's being, the metaphor "God," the image without knowledge of the metaphor, we could be guilty of idolatry, of substituting our own creation of God for the one true and living God. Metaphor may save us from idolatry.

Or look at another of the root metaphors of Christianity and maybe the defining metaphor: Incarnation. I'm fascinated by the fact that Incarnation, prior to its doctrinal function, is first and foremost one of the great and defining examples of what a metaphor is and how it works—and this, not as a thing in the head, but as the root of practice and the shaping of a life. Incarnation claims the identity of Jesus with God, a man from the world of human beings is identified with the divine, with God's own being. This is a central and defining affirmation of Christianity, but it is also a metaphor; and much, if not all of Christian theology through the ages comes through the extension, the ramification, of this root metaphor. The doctrine proclaims that "Jesus is God." But Jesus is clearly a human being, and not the invisible, unknowable creator of the universe. But, as with all metaphors, the claim that Jesus is God, while clearly at one level false, tells us much of what we need to know about God.

In "The Dry Salvages" from *Four Quartets* (1943), T. S. Eliot points to this metaphorical tension between the man and God, between the eternal and the temporal:

> But to apprehend
> The point of intersection of the timeless
> With time, is an occupation for the saint—
> No occupation either, but something given
> And taken, in a lifetime's death in love,
> Ardour and selflessness and self surrender.
> For most of us there is only the unattended
> Moment....
> These are only hints and guesses,
> Hints followed by guesses; and the rest
> Is prayer, observance, discipline, thought and action.
> The hint half guessed, the gift half understood, is
> Incarnation.
> Here the impossible union
> Of spheres of existence is actual.
> (Eliot, 1943, V. 200–207, 212–217)

But Eliot also points out that one of the consequences of the metaphor of Incarnation is not only a mental, cognitive event, it is the expression of the metaphor in life: the working out of a person's spiritual life in practice, "prayer, observance, discipline, thought, and action." The doctrine of the Incarnation, explored as metaphor and not an authoritative requirement, is embodied in practice. This is the working out of the richness of our root metaphors, not an infinite regress, but a progress of ramification in intellect and in practice. And this is the realm of the spiritual director: "What are the implications for your life of the metaphors that guide your journey?"

Some Final Thoughts

As he concluded his lectures on language and metaphor, I. A. Richards (2001 [1936]) asked himself and his audience this question about belief:

> Must we believe what an utterance says if we are to understand it fully? Does the *Divine Comedy*, or the Bible tell us something which we must accept as true if we are to read it aright? These are questions that we cannot possibly answer satisfactorily unless we are clear as to the ways in which metaphoric utterances may say or tell us something. Mr. Eliot remarks somewhere of the *Divine Comedy* that the whole poem is one vast metaphor. It is. And, if so, what is it that we might believe in it? Or is the belief required no more than a readiness to feel and will and live, in certain respects, in accordance with the resultant meaning in so far as we apprehend that meaning—or rather in so far as that meaning apprehends, grasps, takes control of us?
>
> (pp. 90–91)

A personal note, if I may, about belief. I worry at times that all this talk about metaphor may be seen as another liberal, or neo-liberal, way to avoid deep conviction and belief. Am I substituting metaphor for the God I wish to worship? I don't think so. After all, all human language is built on metaphor, literalism merely being a state in which we can no longer recognize that an idea or word or phrase is a metaphor because it has lost its magical, associative character and hardened into literalism.

And I have come to believe that metaphor is at the heart of God's work in the world. John the Evangelist begins his Gospel with the assertion, "In the beginning was the Word" (I:1). Thus Jesus is the language by which God speaks to the creation and its inhabitants. And if, as Richards (2001 [1936]) says, all language is built up of layers and layers of metaphor, then language is metaphor. So we can paraphrase John's opening as, "In the beginning was the Metaphor." The Word of God is the metaphor of Incarnation. Sallie McFague (1982) speaks of Jesus as a parable. I would argue that Jesus is the metaphor, *the* metaphor, the metaphor incarnate, lived. And thus, metaphor becomes the principle of God's speaking in the world; not simply a skill for spiritual directors, but the very meat of spiritual direction.

What if we were to ask ourselves the question, "Am I willing to die for my metaphors?" Am I willing to give my life for the mystery that lies behind the contradictory juxtapositions of truth and falsehood, of sense and nonsense? I, personally, find that, at least in my speculative heart, I am more willing to die for my metaphors than for a set of assertions that I am expected to accept as literarily true, but that fill me with anxiety and doubt. This idea of metaphor has released me from my own vestiges of literalism, the terrible trap of "Do you believe in God?" Yes I do, or no I don't. Metaphor has allowed me to live in the mystery, and give myself in love to a loving God who I know isn't limited by what I project onto the screen labeled "God."

References

Dante Allighieri. (1949). *The Divine Comedy 1: Hell* (D. L. Sayers, Trans.). Penguin. (Original work published 1320.)

Eliot, T. S. (1943). *Four Quartets*. Harcourt.

Fiumara, G. C. (1995). *The Metaphoric Process: Connections between Language and Life*. Routledge.

Geary, J. (2011). *I is an Other*. Harper Collins.

McFague, S. (1982). *Metaphorical Theology: Models of God in Religious Language*. Fortress.

Polanski, R. (director), Towne, R. (Writer), Evans, R. (Producer). (1974). *Chinatown* [film]. Long Road Productions; Robert Evans Company.

Richards, I. A. (2001). *The Philosophy of Rhetoric* (J. Constable, Ed.). Routledge. (Original work published 1936.)

Saint John of the Cross. (1991). *The Collected Works of St. John of the Cross* (K. Kavanaugh and O. Rodriguez, Trans.). Institute of Carmelite Studies Publications.

Soskice, J. M. (1985). *Metaphor and Religious Language.* Clarendon Press.

Shakespeare, W. (2016). *Romeo and Juliet.* B. Mowat and P. Werstine (Eds.). Available at: https://www.folger.edu/explore/shakespeares-works/romeo-and-juliet/read/2/2/ (Original work published 1597).

The Book of Common Prayer, According to the use of The Episcopal Church. (1978). Church Publishing Incorporated.

Tillich, P. (1957). *Dynamics of Faith.* Harper and Row.

Tracy, D. (1975). *Blessed Rage for Order.* Seabury.

Tracy, D. (1979). Metaphor and Religion: The Test Case of Christian Texts. In S. Sacks, (Ed.) *On Metaphor.* (pp. 89–104). University of Chicago Press.

Chapter 5

Radical Love, Liberation, and Justice

For Self and Others

Katherine E. Kirby

It was nine or ten years ago that an incredible therapist introduced me to the work of Thich Nhat Hanh, through the book *Peace Is Every Step* (1991). In the years prior, several difficult circumstances in my life had awakened an anxiety that gripped me tightly. Though I was seemingly functioning well, and I thought I was handling the stress, I would come home from work and my dear three-year-old dog would run to me with excitement… and promptly throw up. The poor thing was absorbing the waves of anxiety coursing through me. My canary in the coalmine. In truth, I was profoundly struggling, and this amazing therapist helped me find my way. After several years of work together, it was during the year leading up to his retirement that he introduced engaged mindfulness in a way that opened up a new pathway for me. Little did I know that this path would eventually lead to one of the most powerful and joyful teaching experiences of my career. I offer this chapter as a reflection on my experience of creating and teaching a course on Engaged Buddhism, as well as an encouragement to others to forge into vulnerable, transformative, and powerful spaces that merge intellectual inquiry with emotional and spiritual exploration in the classroom. I hope that this chapter can offer readers a way to think about how this kind of engaged spiritual exploration reflects the aims and some of the methods of group spiritual direction.

A Pathway from Wilderness to Shared Exploration

Let me begin by explaining the path that led me to create my "Radical Love, Liberation, and Justice" course for undergraduate students at Saint Michael's College near Burlington, Vermont. My own spiritual practice had deepened in unexpected ways when the COVID-19 pandemic hit in 2020. Like many people, I found myself struggling with some intense grief, anxiety, and fear of all kinds. A friend of mine from high school, Reggie Hubbard, began teaching yoga on Zoom, and I was there in a heartbeat. His professional work at the time was in the realm of politics—including advocacy, activism, organizing work—and because of this orientation, his yoga classes were connected to real things happening in the world, and real vulnerabilities we were all feeling,

DOI: 10.4324/9781003742852-5

in a way I had never seen before. For example, he would talk us through deep belly breathing into the grief and fear we were all feeling in the face of an illness that was stealing people's ability to breathe. As COVID raged, misinformation about the supposed Chinese origins of the virus fed pandemic anxiety and fueled prejudice, and as a result, people were being targeted by anti-Asian bigotry, violence, and hate. Then, on May 25th, 2020, George Floyd was murdered by police, and people across the world took to the streets to protest. These yoga classes became spaces of community, dialogue, critical thinking, reflection, social critique, and processing anger and sadness and fear together, during which we were deeply feeling and exploring our own psychological, emotional, spiritual selves as we responded to what was happening in the world.[1]

At the same time, Thich Nhat Hanh's community in Plum Village shifted all of their retreats to synchronous online format, so I was able to practice with, and learn from, the monks, nuns, and lay teachers taught by Zen master Thich Nhat Hanh (1926–2022), who is often credited as playing a significant role in bringing Buddhism to the West. Created in 1982, Plum Village was the first of the retreat centers founded by Thich Nhat Hanh for the practice of engaged Buddhism and mindful living.[2] As I learned more about his relationship with Rev. Dr. Martin Luther King, Jr., his radical protest during the Vietnam War, and his teachings on contemporary problems and activism today, I found in Thich Nhat Hanh's Plum Village tradition a powerful alignment and grounding for my yoga practice that felt both personally freeing and empowering for responsible social justice action.

During this time, I took every opportunity that came my way to be part of online workshops, talks, and conversations that were focused on the critique of any "wellness work" that encourages "spiritual bypassing"—a sidestepping of the difficult, deep work of personal examination and/or social transformation. As I will discuss in more depth below, this concept of "spiritual bypassing" was introduced by John Welwood in his essay, "Principles of Inner Work: Psychological and Spiritual" (1984). As applied to yoga, meditation, and mindfulness spaces, this critique identifies that so much of the "wellness work" we see today ends up promoting a kind of escapism that avoids or suppresses painful emotion and evades accountability and responsibility for social change. The alternative is a practice that has the potential for deep spiritual healing and powerful interconnection that compels us to action for a better, more just world. Such practice, I realized more deeply, was a pathway to a radical love, a radical liberation, and radical justice.

Before long, my community-engaged learning partner and I had to decide to pause our partnership in a course where my students work with elders at an assisted living home in Burlington, because COVID made our work together too dangerous and too difficult. Faced with the need to replace that seminar course, I knew that I wanted to create a new course that would engage students in exploring this work that I had found so compelling. When

I told my yoga teacher the idea, he said, "We are in a liminal space. You have to do it. Trust me." That was all I needed to hear, and the stack of books that I had been wanting to read on the integration of Buddhism, mindfulness, meditation, and yoga with radical racial justice work was winging its way to me that very same afternoon.

The first iteration of the course was completely on Zoom, and I was blown away by the conversations we were having. A couple of months into the semester, at a faculty and staff lunch, my friend and colleague in Counseling Services at the college, asked about the course. She told me that she had heard about it from several (unnamed) students during their counseling sessions—where they were drawing on ideas and conversations from our course. In class discussions throughout the semester, students described feeling more space and flexibility with their feelings, and they shared insights into obstacles and struggles they encounter in their own inner work and in their relationships. When registration happened for the second (in-person) iteration, it was full within 15 minutes, and within about an hour, I had 25 petitions to join the course over the cap. There has been similar demand every time I have offered the course. It has also led to co-creating a weekend retreat called "Finding Calm: An Interfaith Retreat on Mindfulness, Meditation, and Prayer," with a colleague who is Catholic. The message became clear: Students were—and are—hungry for space and guidance in exploring the spiritual dimensions of their lives and their role in their communities and society. In teaching this course, and in conversations with colleagues and spiritual directors, I have come to more deeply understand the power of creating space for students to engage in a practice paralleling spiritual direction—a space for which many of us in higher education realize our students have been calling.

Course Aims and Purpose

The particular texts, films, and resources that I find useful are unique to my own approach; but they may offer inspiration in your own course design.

My vision for this Engaged Buddhism course grew directly out of the pathway my own practice had taken, and thus had a two-fold aim. First, a huge number of students at Saint Michael's College are social justice oriented. They want the world to be more just and equitable and compassionate, and they want to be a part of creating that. The College's founding order—the Society of Saint Edmund—has a long history of work for equity and justice, especially racial justice. Our students, however, don't always connect the justice they seek with the *radical liberation* necessary for justice, especially their own self-liberation. The Indigenous Australian visual artist, activist, and academic Lilla Watson articulates this beautifully, saying, "If you have come to help me, you are wasting your time. But if you have come because your liberation is bound up with mine, then let us work together."[3] I view collective liberation, and what that means about freeing my own mind and heart from socialization and indoctrination into white supremacy, to be a crucial part of my work. Following the murder of George Floyd in 2020 and that summer of protest, students seemed to be yearning for racial justice with an intensity that, for many of them, was new. So, one primary aim for the course was engaging students in a robust dive into work on engaged Buddhism and collective liberation, wherein each of us must seek our own liberation and collective liberation for all.

The second part of my two-fold aim for the course was to respond to what I see as a yearning within our students for a deeper, richer, and more nourishing spiritual life—something beyond the materialistic, consumeristic, social media-dominant world so many of us inhabit. College students are seeking support in their struggles with anxiety, depression, and other mental health challenges at unprecedented levels. In fact, *so many of us* are suffering in these ways. I see and feel a deep yearning underneath this suffering, and a sadness, a grief, a hopelessness—compounded by a frustration because we can't find relief, or we don't know how to find what feels missing. My second aim, therefore, is to engage students in a semester of dialogue and exploration of both their relationship with Others in our suffering world and their relationship with their own suffering selves.

The guiding questions we explore in the course are among the most vital and transformative: What does it mean to seek and cultivate *radical love, radical liberation*, and *radical justice*, for yourself and for others? What does it mean to deeply and radically love, nurture, and have compassion for yourself? What does it mean to love other people in that way? What does it mean to seek radical liberation, or radical freedom, for yourself? Liberation from what? What does it mean to seek such liberation for others? What does it mean to create radical justice in our world, so filled with suffering, and violence, and—sometimes possibly worse—indifference? Exploring these questions with students has been one of the most powerful experiences in my career.

Fundamental questions about love, freedom, justice, and meaning may come up in a range of academic courses. We likely wrestle with them in our personal therapeutic work. And they surely arise in our spiritual practices. However, the connections between these core human phenomena and how they manifest in the intellectual, psychological, emotional, and spiritual dimensions of our lives is too rarely made the central focus of intentional space. It is in diving into such exploration together that this course comes to reflect many aspects of group spiritual direction.

Through readings, films, individual research projects connected to their majors, and cultivation of a personal practice of some kind, the course seeks to help students understand the radical power of mindfulness for personal and social/collective liberation. This framework is informed by Reverend angel Kyodo williams' explanation of "radical" in *Radical Dharma: Talking Race, Love, and Liberation*, co-authored with Lama Rod Owens and Jasmine Syedullah. Rev. angel[4] offers a definition of radical as "relating to or affecting the fundamental nature of something; far reaching or thorough… going *to the root*" (williams, 2016, p. xix). We are seeking the fundamental nature—the root—of love, liberation, and justice. After exploring this broadly, we examine recent applications to racial liberation and racial justice work.

Course Design and Approach

It is important to acknowledge that I am not a Dharma teacher, and I do not claim expertise in Buddhism. Also, although I recognize the resonances, I am not attempting to offer my students spiritual direction in the sense of explicitly directing them. My training is in philosophy, and I approach the material I've chosen for the course as a philosopher and a teacher, in alignment with Paulo Freire's analysis in *Pedagogy of the Oppressed* (Freire, 1993 [1970]), where students and teachers are studying texts and asking questions *together*, learning from each other as we share our insights, lived experience, and interpretations with one another, and in this course, cultivating our own practices of meditation, yoga, and/or mindfulness. This course is philosophical and interdisciplinary, and it draws students from a wide variety of majors because it fulfills a Junior Seminar requirement in our core curriculum. In my approach, philosophical inquiry requires self-examination and phenomenological reflection on lived experience, and this fundamentally engages the spiritual dimension of our lives.

The themes of the course, which I will explain further below, emerge in each of the texts we engage. My course design centers on four main texts, supplemented by films, videos, student research, and meditation practice. We begin the semester with a unit on Engaged Buddhism. We start by watching interviews with Thich Nhat Hanh so that they can hear and feel his presence and way of being in the world, and we then read a selection of chapters from the Parallax Press collection *True Peace Work: Essential Writings on Engaged Buddhism* (2019). In this three-week unit, we study together the writings of Dharma teachers and practitioners including Thich Nhat Hanh, Sulak Sivaraksa, Jack Kornfield, Kenneth Kraft, Zenju Earthlyn Manuel, bell hooks, and the Dalai Lama. Each week unfolds one of our core themes, and we integrate segments of recorded Dharma talks and *Walk with Me* (Francis and Pugh, 2017), a powerful film about Plum Village. We then move to a unit on *The Book of Joy: Lasting Happiness in a Changing World* (Dalai Lama, Tutu, and Abrams, 2016), which is a fascinating and funny account of the conversations that took place between His Holiness the Dalai Lama and Archbishop Desmond Tutu, collected by Douglas Abrams during a visit in Dharamsala for the Dalai Lama's 80th birthday. We first learn about each of their lives and work through two films. *Children of the Light* (Engle, 2014) explains the history of Apartheid and Desmond Tutu's incredible resistance and leadership, and *Road to Peace* (Stuparich, 2012) describes the Dalai Lama's exile and work for peace in the world. Our course themes again emerge through *The Book of Joy's* exploration of the possibility of finding joy even in the face of terrible suffering and oppression. Students love this book and the tender, warm, funny friendship that can be felt through their words. Our third major unit applies engaged Buddhism to racial liberation and racial justice. There are many exceptional recent books on this topic. I find *Radical Dharma: Talking Race, Love, and Liberation* (williams, Owens, and Syedullah, 2016), a text mentioned above, to be among the very best. Our same core themes emerge once again, this time through the exploration of intersectional collective liberation that Rev. angel, Lama Rod, and Jasmine Syedullah offer. We supplement the text with a TEDx Talk and a presentation in a church delivered by Rev. angel Kyodo williams (williams, 2017, 2019). We then read selected chapters from Lama Rod's *Love and Rage: The Path of Liberation through Anger* (Owens, 2020) and watch several online conversations with him. Student research presentations on engaged Buddhism connected to their majors and/or minors constitute our fourth unit, which offers students a chance to connect what they have learned to something important to them, personally. These research projects consistently blow me away, and they offer all of us a glimpse into the many additional dimensions and applications of practice that could be explored. Finally, we conclude our semester by watching together the film *Fierce Light: When Spirit Meets Action* (2008) by filmmaker Velcrow Ripper. The film's main theme aligns beautifully with our course themes, as it explores global movements that invest activism with spirituality.

My teaching approach in this course is Socratic in that our classroom conversations are generated by questions about human experience, and we offer our interpretations, ideas, questions, and critiques, in dialogue with one another and the texts we have read or videos we have watched in preparation for the day's discussion. On most class days, prior to class, students have read an assigned text and/or watched an assigned video or film, and they have submitted either a short reflection essay or a short paragraph. Sometimes I give them specific guiding questions to answer, and sometimes I simply ask, "What did you find compelling, powerful, interesting, confusing, controversial, and/or problematic in the text/video?" Although such assignments every class period require substantial grading time for me, two important benefits outweigh that challenge. First, students are ready and eager to talk in class. Second, students will share and process things in these small written assignments that they do not feel comfortable sharing in class. Because of the spiritual and emotional dimension of their work in this course, it's important for them to have this avenue of communication with me. My feedback can create dialogue with them individually, to supplement the group dialogue of class sessions.

Importantly, at the start of every class session, we begin with meditation together. I most often utilize online meditations led by trained teachers, from sites such as *Insight Timer*, so that students learn about resources that are accessible to them. Occasionally, I will lead them in a meditation I have learned, or we will meditate silently outside. I carefully select each day's meditation just prior to the class session in alignment with what they have read or watched in preparation for class and what we discussed in the prior class session, as this creates continuity and inspiration for the day's discussion. Occasionally, I select a meditation based on what I sense is the vibe in the room, particularly at times of the semester when they are more intensely stressed, overwhelmed with work, or reacting to difficult things happening on campus or in the world.

I find this meditative practice together to be essential for three main reasons. First, it brings all of us into the present moment and into our time together, leaving outside pressures and stressors outside of our 95 minutes, to the degree that is possible. Second, students are required to cultivate a practice of their own outside of class, experimenting with different modalities (e.g., meditation, yoga, etc.), and for those who are having difficulty finding what works for them, this group practice ensures they have some time feeling the benefits of practice and some exposure to different kinds of practice. Third, the meditations I choose integrate the topics of the day's discussion in a way that is different from reading texts and watching videos—an embodied engagement that guides them in checking in with their own selves, spiritually, emotionally, and physically, not just intellectually.

We then begin our class discussion. Most often, I put them into small groups to discuss the reading and assignment they have prepared. Because our texts address themes that are often challenging emotionally and in our personal lives, this small group forum provides a space that allows for a bit more vulnerability, building an environment of support. Following this, we open up the conversation for a whole-group discussion. I first act as a scribe, organizing their ideas on the board in a way that allows me to integrate the conversation into a cohesive picture of the key ideas in our texts and pose questions for them to ponder as they move on to the next reading and assignment. I always have in mind the ideas, understandings, and questions that I want us to hold by the end of the class session, but I find it essential that students have the freedom to express what they find compelling, confusing, fascinating, or problematic in our texts. Indeed, I believe it would be a problematic hypocrisy if a course about the power and necessity of liberation did not allow for students' passions and interests to generate and co-determine the substance and direction of each conversation. It can be challenging to allow our examination to unfold in this way, but it is also thrilling. It never fails to keep me thinking in new ways and learning, myself. And most importantly, it is an opportunity for me to guide them in empowering themselves to bravely and responsibly undertake the intellectual, emotional, and spiritual journey of collaborative, dialogic learning and meaning-making.

Three times during the semester, we integrate conversation about their own practice, as we have an assignment category that requires that they cultivate a regular practice of their choosing and keep a journal. I do not require that they write about every activity that they do, because I do not want their practice to be reduced to just an assignment that they tick off each day. I want them to be able to just be present as they practice—and knowing that they have to do something with the activity afterward contradicts that way of engaging. Rather, I encourage them to explore, experiment, and try new modalities throughout the week, and, at some point during their week, spend a little time writing about how their practice is going. I assign a journal prompt just before I collect them, only three times during the semester, and I grade them based only on completion and thoughtfulness, not on accuracy or particular details. I offer feedback that encourages them and mentions connections to our texts and discussion for their continued thinking.

As our semester winds down, students select a topic for their independent research that connects to their major or other academic passions. I organize them into small groups of three to six students based on those choices, and they utilize academic journal articles or book chapters and other sources appropriate to their sub-topic to learn as much as they can in a couple of weeks. Each student presents, integrating our course themes, and the group is responsible for leading the discussion for approximately half of the class session, including selecting or leading a meditation. I am always incredibly impressed by these projects and presentations, and students show such passion and enthusiasm for sharing what they have learned.

At the conclusion of the semester, students submit a final paper that asks them to explain the most important things they have learned about radical love for self and for others, radical liberation for self and for others, and radical justice for all. They integrate course texts and films of their choosing (with some guidelines for selecting), their research, and their own practice to explore their ideas, insights, and continued questioning of self-reflection. Most importantly, this assignment is designed to offer them one more opportunity to think through the themes of our course, reflect on their own practice and experience, and express what impacted them most powerfully intellectually, emotionally, and spiritually.

Core Themes of the Course

The main themes of the course arise in each unit, as the texts, films, and videos I have chosen engage our main questions, though from different angles. It is not possible to capture everything we discuss in a semester, and of course, this changes in response to the unique group of students that find their way to the course each semester. In what follows, I offer examples of how our themes emerge and a snapshot of how I endeavor to guide students through their own self-reflective exploration.

The Critique of Spiritual Bypassing

As I note above, one of the first things we consider in our course is the current critique of "wellness work" that encourages spiritual bypassing, which is a sidestepping of the difficult, deep work of personal or social examination. John Welwood coined the term in 1984, which he explains in a 2011 interview in *Tricycle: The Buddhist Review*, as follows:

> Spiritual bypassing… describe[s] a process I saw happening in the Buddhist community I was in, and also in myself. Although most of us were sincerely trying to work on ourselves, I noticed a widespread tendency to use spiritual ideas and practices to sidestep or avoid facing unresolved emotional issues, psychological wounds, and unfinished developmental tasks. When we are spiritually bypassing, we often use the goal of awakening or liberation to try to rise above the raw and messy side of our humanness before we have fully faced and made peace with it.
>
> (Fossella, 2011, n.p.)

There are practitioners today who are powerfully exploring the ways in which this kind of spiritual bypassing applies to social justice issues, suggesting that we are likewise bypassing the hard, painful work of deeply understanding our complicity in injustice and inequity, and thus we are avoiding taking responsibility for action to effect social change. Wellness work can become escapism both personally and socially, and the latter is a failure to recognize that thriving as a human being requires a deep compassion and responsibility for others. This is my starting point for the course because, in my experience, students are quite unsatisfied with shallow versions of wellness work that purport to offer a solution to the profound pain, sadness, and anger they feel, both personally and in the face of social injustice, violence, and inequity. Introducing this critique of spiritual bypassing guides them in understanding the crucial move of embracing the incredibly difficult and messy work involved in radical liberation work, for self and others.

Interbeing, Hungry Ghosts, Loving Compassion, Sangha, and the Work of Liberation

In our first unit, selected essays from *True Peace Work* (2019) challenge students' pre-conceptions of Buddhism and mindfulness as a purely personal, self-focused practice.[5] In an essay entitled "Buddhism in a World of Change," Sulak Sivaraksa (2019, p. 88) says, "Many people, particularly in the West, think that Buddhism is only for deep meditation and personal transformation, that it has nothing to do with society. This is not true." Students often find his article compelling, as he goes on to explain how Buddhism can, and *must*, invest society with values and principles that combat poverty, violence, war, economic inequality, and suffering. We find further discussion of the necessity of engagement with the world in Thich Nhat Hanh's "Why We Need a Global Ethic," where he contends:

> If Buddhism is not engaged, it's not real Buddhism. This is the attitude of the bodhisattvas, beings whose whole intention and actions are to relieve suffering. We practice meditation and mindfulness not only for ourselves; we practice to relieve the suffering of all beings and of the Earth. With the insight of interbeing—that we are elementally interconnected with all other beings—we know that when other people suffer less, we suffer less. And when we suffer less, other people suffer less.
>
> (Hanh, 2019c, p. 297)

Video interviews with Thich Nhat Hanh bring this explanation to life for students as we learn about the protests that he and fellow monks and nuns staged during the Vietnam War, as well as their work to address poverty and inequity, and their recent work on environmental responsibility. Our class discussions reveal that students find the notion of *interbeing* compelling and applicable to the social, political, economic, environmental, religious, and ethical issues that matter the most to them. Our initial readings point us toward a more radical love and compassion and a more radical orientation toward justice and liberation.

Once students have become intrigued by the critique of spiritual bypassing and this introduction to Engaged Buddhism, we then turn to the question of how our culture trains us as humans. We ask: from what must we be liberated? We read several pieces that explore the way our society and culture teach us—indoctrinate us, really—to always be running, to see our value and worth in how "productive" we are. In many sources, Thich Nhat Hanh talks about how there is so much noise—all around us, and also within our minds. In "Suffering Is Not Enough" Thich Nhat Hanh reflects,

> We are so busy we hardly have time to look at the people we love, even in our own household, and to look at ourselves. Society is organized in a way that even when we have some leisure time, we don't know how to use it to get back in touch with ourselves.... We are not used to being with ourselves, and we act as if we don't like ourselves and are trying to escape from ourselves.
>
> (Hanh, 2019b, p. 5)

We run, run, run as if we're chasing something—or perhaps as if we are being chased. Together, we think through what he says about no longer running. For our in-class meditation on the days we discuss this topic, we watch short videos from Plum Village and we practice mindful walking, or slow-walking, outside together. We talk about what it's like—what they notice both outside of them and inside of them—when they practice mindful walking in the days that follow. What is this practice like on their way to class, to the gym or dining hall, when they're with friends, and in other times? We use the physical practice of slow, mindful walking to guide our self-reflection and discussion on what it means to be *running* all of the time spiritually, mentally, and emotionally. This resonates *deeply* with students, as we consider the impact that constant rushing and pressure has on our inner lives.

We follow this with several articles from *True Peace Work* on community and what happens when our community or society fails to take care of people. In "Community as a Resource," Thich Nhat Hanh explains,

> In Buddhist mythology, a hungry ghost is a wandering soul whose throat is too narrow for food or drink to pass through. Hungry ghosts need love, but they do not have the capacity to receive it.... What they really need is something to take refuge in.
>
> (Hanh, 2019a, p. 230)

This, too, is an explanation that hits home for a lot of students, and I always tread lightly during these days of class. Students write about relating painfully to this concept of the "hungry ghost," and a few muster the courage to share those thoughts in class discussion. We consider whether some degree of this condition grows in each of us as we are socialized into our hyper-individualistic culture, and we hold space for sadness that emerges as we contemplate this.

This leads us into powerful discussions about profound love and compassion for self and for others. As painful emotions emerge in students' reading, writing, and class discussion, we watch and discuss a segment of a Dharma Talk[6] from Thich Nhat Hanh that includes a teaching on the seeds within us. He explains that there are all kinds of seeds that exist in our stored consciousness: seeds of fear, sadness, anger, joy, patience, love, compassion, discrimination, non-discrimination, etc. When these seeds are triggered, they become mental formations that fill our minds and hearts. Here, he discusses how we can recognize and tenderly embrace those feelings as they arrive, and breathe enough space into ourselves to let them be. In class we talk about this capacity we have to release our grip on our emotions and thereby no longer *be gripped* and controlled by them. And in that gentler space, Thay[7] tells us, we can be curious and ask what the feeling is about, and gain insight. We can let the feeling be present and pass through. In this Dharma Talk and in "Community as a Resource" (Hanh, 2019a), he offers us the practice of the 5-year-old-self meditation, where we recognize that the feelings we have are likely very old, and we can respond to our small selves with loving tenderness and care we need.[8] Further, we consider his suggestion that we can do this for others, even those we perceive as enemies—recognizing the five-year-old within them who is suffering, and thereby causing suffering. Here, mindfulness practice meets psychology and phenomenology of emotion and suffering. Students love the idea of relating to their own young selves in this way, realizing their capacity for a more profound compassion for themselves, on the whole and in moments of powerful and painful emotion. They also see the tremendous value of turning this practice toward others.

However, its application to those we perceive as enemies, or those who have done harm to us, always leads to challenging conversations in class about forgiveness, accountability, and responsibility. We add two essays from *True Peace Work* (2019) by the Dalai Lama, "Genuine Compassion" and "Hope for the Future: 1988." In the former, he talks about how we might shift to be angry at the anger inside our enemy—an anger that has gripped our enemy and is motivating their harmful action, an anger within them from which they have not yet escaped. He says,

> When you train your mind in this way, gradually you will be able to extend your compassion toward all living creatures, including your enemy… I can change my own mental attitude, and it brings me some real joy and inner strength.
>
> (Dalai Lama, 2019a, p. 157)

We consider the idea that forgiveness may be more about the liberation of one who forgives, and we do a deep dive into philosophical examination of forgiveness and what it requires and enacts. This is a tremendously vulnerable space, as students reflect on their own wounds and relationships, and these conversations require a great deal of care, caution, and direction. At this and many other moments in the course, I remind students to be their own gatekeepers, carefully choosing what they wish to share. And I remind them to take very seriously their classmates' right to privacy and need for sensitivity. Ultimately, I aim to guide the conversation toward the small glimmer of freedom we might begin to see when we realize that we can choose how we move through each of our days, activities, and emotional responses, and we consider how the individual practice they will cultivate during the semester can be guided by more compassion and love and care for themselves and others.

Our readings tell us that a Sangha characterized by compassion and love can offer us the refuge we need and support in our vulnerability. For Buddhists, *Sangha*—along with the Dharma and Buddha Nature—is part of the Three Jewels. Thich Nhat Hanh (2019a, p. 231) calls Sangha a "spiritual family", and says:

> Taking refuge in a Sangha means putting your trust in a community of solid members who practice mindfulness together. It is difficult if not impossible to practice mindfulness without a Sangha. Teachers and teachings are important for the practice, but a community of friends is the most essential ingredient.
>
> (Hanh, 2019a, p. 227)

We read this in the context of exploring what our culture tends to do to us—the dislocation and the severing from our own self and from others—and how the cultivation of true community can heal this. Zenju Earthlyn Manuel's

"Where the Heart Lives" (2019) offers us a beautiful and heart-wrenching explanation of how systems of oppression in the US, and experiences of being unloved or abused or neglected or rejected or ignored, render people homeless—that is, seeking some kind of refuge. Manuel then explains how *Sangha*—or a community of love and care—can offer this. Manuel shares:

> [O]ur spiritual communities must be sanctuaries that understand the depth at which people have been stripped of their culture for a more dominant one. In sanctuary, we recover from being lost and take refuge in shared community, the collective embodiment of all that symbolizes home.
>
> (Manuel, 2019, p. 263)

Manuel relates *interbeing* to Dr. Martin Luther King Jr.'s "beloved community," and the "single garment of destiny" that he so famously described.

This reading is paired with "Toward a Worldwide Culture of Love," by bell hooks. In this piece, she helps us think about how capitalism, consumerism, and systems of oppression create a culture of domination that devalues—and actually cannot co-exist with—real love (hooks, 2019, p. 332). She speaks of how this devaluing culture creates a wound in the heart and a wound in the collective. This wound too often causes people who are fighting for liberation and justice to drag mindsets of domination into that work. She explains:

> To work for peace and justice, we begin with the individual practice of love, because it is there that we can experience firsthand love's transformative power… If we grow into our adult years without knowing how to love, how then can we create social movements that will end domination, exploitation, and oppression?
>
> (hooks, 2019, p. 323)

Here, we introduce very directly our course's application of Engaged Buddhism to racial justice and collective liberation, beginning with self-reflective discussion about how this culture of domination wounds us and prevents the radical kind of love we have been discussing. We examine the ways we are enculturated into domination mindsets, and we think through why love cannot co-exist with domination. We return to the idea that the radical "transformative power" of love can, and must, work to create radical collective liberation and justice.

Ubuntu, Compassion, Forgiveness, and Finding Liberation and Joy in the Face of Suffering

As we shift to our second unit, the main themes of the course emerge in new ways as we read *The Book of Joy* (Dalai Lama, Tutu, and Abrams, 2016). Our class discussions on this text philosophically explore the nature of what they call the eight "obstacles to joy" and the eight "pillars of joy," drawing on both our lived experience and our knowledge of other philosophers and thinkers from other disciplines. We consider what it would mean to invest social justice work with the deep kind of joy—which is different from happiness and, according to Archbishop Tutu and the Dalai Lama, is possible even in the throes of tremendous suffering. Significantly, we wrestle with their suggestion that the kind of wellness, or healing, that we seek for ourselves is simply not possible in isolation from the suffering of the world.

We begin by meeting Archbishop Desmond Tutu and the Dalai Lama through film, so that students can picture these two spiritual leaders as they read their words. We watch *Children of the Light* (Engle, 2014), which tells the story of Apartheid in South Africa, and Archbishop Tutu's work for liberation and reconciliation, in all of its complexity and imperfection. We then watch *Road to Peace* (Stuparich, 2012), which tells the story of the Dalai Lama's exile and follows him as he meets with and works with a variety of people and communities. In our class discussions about these films, we wrestle with the messiness of social justice and liberation work. The films reveal intense human suffering and we spend time considering together how the process of addressing this suffering uncovers deep wounds and often does not result in complete or perfect resolution. The films also reveal the possibility of holding both intense woundedness and intense calm, hope, and even joy, demonstrated by these two leaders. So many of us find it difficult to hold both realities at the same time, and most students leave these films wanting to hear more. This offers us the perfect entry point into the conversations between the Dalai Lama and Desmond Tutu in *The Book of Joy* (Dalai Lama, Tutu, and Abrams, 2016), aimed at finding joy even in the midst of so much suffering. They describe a joy rooted in the kind of radical love for self and others that we explored in our previous unit—a capacity within the self for compassion that, if missing, renders us less human and less free.

Early on, the Dalai Lama explains "Our whole society has a materialistic culture… [and in this] way of life, there's no concept of friendship, no concept of love, just work, twenty-four hours a day, like a machine" (Dalai Lama, Tutu, and Abrams, 2016, p. 127). Students easily recognize the connection to what Thich Nhat Hanh described as frenzied living, or the aforementioned running, running, running through life. Archbishop Tutu agrees with this indictment of our society, and their discussion leads us to identify and critique the aspects of our own lives that are driven by materialism, consumption, and unconscious competitiveness and over-valuing of work. Once again, we are also faced with the individualism we are taught to value in our society.

Through his explanation of *interbeing*, Thich Nhat Hanh had given us an alternative, explaining that we are radically interconnected, with our lives interwoven and impacting each other. In *Children of the Light* (Engle, 2014) and *The Book of Joy* (Dalai Lama, Tutu, and Abrams, 2016, p. 60), we learn from Archbishop Tutu about *Ubuntu*: "A person is a person through other persons… we are bound up together. We are bound up and can be human only together." We consider together this fundamental shift in the way we might think about what it means to be a human person. We explore the possibility of honoring the uniqueness and irreplaceability of each person while likewise recognizing that each person is who they are because of their relationships. I select meditations to start our class sessions that encourage us to feel our interdependence and connection to others, both loved ones and strangers. Here, we return to our core theme of the necessity of conscientious and responsible engagement with the world. Early in *The Book of Joy*, Archbishop Tutu says, "It's how we are made. I mean we are wired to be compassionate… We are wired to be caring for the other and generous to one another. We shrivel when we are not able to interact" (Dalai Lama, Tutu, and Abrams, 2016, p. 59). He goes on to explain, "we flourish in community. When we become self-centered, turning in on ourselves, as sure as anything, we are going to find one day a deep, deep *deep* frustration" (Dalai Lama, Tutu, and Abrams, 2016, p. 62). In class discussion, students express great interest in the idea that compassion and generosity are a fundamental part of our human nature, not just the self-interest that our culture seems to encourage. We ask about this shriveling and deep frustration that he describes, drawing on our own experience and questioning our enculturated beliefs.

The section of the book on "The Obstacles to Joy" (Dalai Lama, Tutu, and Abrams, 2016) offers us explanation of the immensely relatable suffering that takes the form of fear, anxiety, anger, sadness and grief, despair, loneliness, envy, fear of death, and more. As we read this section, I assign a journal prompt that asks students to explore one or two of the obstacles in their own lives, and I collect their journal entries up to that point. What I find is that most students express finding comfort and insight as they compare these chapters with their own experience. When we then turn to the section on "The Pillars of Joy," we discuss the power of perspective, humility, humor, acceptance, forgiveness, gratitude, compassion, and generosity—four pillars of the mind and four pillars of the heart, our authors tell us. I select meditations for our class sessions that tap into these "pillars," and we discuss them not as magic solutions, but rather as capacities we can cultivate as we choose how we will respond to suffering in our lives—capacities that have potentially transformative power.

In every semester I have taught the course, one of the most difficult discussions we have centers around the complexity and difficulty of real forgiveness. This includes asking what forgiveness is and what it requires, and contemplating whether anger can remain and even have value when one forgives. Our discussions explore how forgiveness is, at least in part, a freeing of *ourselves* from the wrongdoing and/or the one who has harmed us. These conversations about forgiveness arise naturally from student reactions to the films and the chapters. I am always incredibly impressed with their ability to think through very thorny questions, grounded in their own lived experience of forgiving and needing to be forgiven. In one semester, for example, a student from Rwanda offered deeply insightful challenges to what the Dalai Lama and Archbishop Tutu suggest, while also acknowledging the liberation that forgiveness can effect. It led to several days of engaged discussion during which we considered arguments for the impossibility of forgiveness. I tread very carefully through these class sessions, as many students offer their own experiences of violence or harm, and as they deeply wrestle with their own desire for freedom from that harm and their own difficulty in forgiving.[9] Opening up this discourse gives students the necessary room to struggle to understand a complex human phenomenon, to compare it against their own experience, to gain insight into their own experience, to hold space to hear and learn from others' experience, and to expand their own understanding or understand forgiveness differently.

Throughout our unit on *The Book of Joy* (Dalai Lama, Tutu, and Abrams, 2016), we frequently discuss the importance of refusing spiritual bypassing and avoiding toxic positivity. Archbishop Tutu and the Dalai Lama are not arguing for the suppression of important emotional responses to the world. Rather, they are offering a possible way of *responding* to our emotional responses that creates greater freedom and allows for joy. We link Thich Nhat Hanh's work with author Douglas Abrams' explanation of Archbishop Tutu's and the Dalai Lama's suggestions. Abrams explains:

> Some might wonder what our own joy has to do with countering injustice and inequality. What does our happiness have to do with addressing the suffering of the world? In short, the more we heal our own pain, the more we can turn to the pain of others. But in a surprising way, what the Archbishop and the Dalai Lama were saying is that the way we heal our own pain is actually by turning to the pain of others. It is a virtuous cycle. The more we turn toward others, the more joy we experience, and the more joy we experience, the more we can bring joy to others.... So being more joyful is not just about having more fun. We're talking about a more empathic, more empowered, even more spiritual state of mind that is totally engaged with the world.
>
> (Dalai Lama, Tutu, and Abrams, 2016, p. 63)

Our class discussions center around the empowerment and liberation that Archbishop Tutu and the Dalai Lama say is possible through radical compassionate action, and the joy that emerges.

Throughout our reading of this text, our collective liberation theme continues to weave—where freedom for self and freedom for others are inextricably bound together. As we prepare to move into our final text unit, I tell them about the work of Stephen (Steve) Bantu Biko, who fought against Apartheid in South Africa and was murdered by jailers. He says in *I Write What I Like*, "The most potent weapon in the hands of the oppressor is the mind of the oppressed" (Biko, 2002 [1978], p. 68). As long as we are mentally unfree, we will continue to serve and reinforce oppressive systems. Biko points to the necessity for every person living in a culture or system characterized by domination or oppression to seek their own mental liberation from it as they seek to create a just and liberated society. This idea leads directly to our final text unit, where we explore applications of our core themes to radical racial liberation and justice.

Broken-Heartedness, Self-Liberation, and Social Revolution for Collective Liberation and Justice

One of the most powerful books that brings together engaged Buddhism and racial liberation work is *Radical Dharma* (williams, Owens, and Syedullah, 2016). The testimony, reflections, and intersectional analysis offered by the authors resonate deeply with students. Our core themes for the course emerge once again. Early on, we find Rev. angel Kyodo williams articulating the necessity of conscientious engagement with the world, saying:

> If the fruit of practice is not a desire to respond to the world, if it just remains in response to your own needs, "me" is all you are seeing: "I want to feel better, I want to feel like a spiritual person. I want to be seen as right. But I don't want to actually be responsible for the world that I'm in." Then you haven't yet woken up.
>
> (williams, 2016, p. xxix).

Mindful living is about awakening, both to one's own inner life and one's place in the reality of the world. *Radical Dharma's* application to racism and racial liberation speaks directly to what our students—and all of us—are experiencing and questioning. It requires that readers see ourselves implicated in structures and systems that are harmful and violent, and embrace responsibility for actively working to resist those systems and create a new society.

In our class discussions, some students find it difficult to understand their own participation in the kinds of oppression this text discusses, but when it clicks for them that their own humanity, healing, and freedom requires responsibility and action for collective liberation for everyone from such systems, a profound shift occurs. We begin by watching together a recording of a talk/homily, called "Unlearning the Ways of the System," that Rev. angel delivered at All Saints Church in Pasadena in 2019. In this talk she integrates US history of racism with the Christian Bible to explain how systems of violence and oppression indoctrinate us. Drawing from scripture, she notes how these systems close our eyes and block our ears and dull our minds. She then pulls on scripture that calls us to "turn around and be healed," applying this to our responsibility to free ourselves from such indoctrination, find liberation for ourselves, and then answer a call to be sent to create a better, freer world (williams, 2019). This initial introduction opens up for us a conversation about the interdependence of our spiritual endeavor for our own well-being, healing, and freedom with our loving engagement with the world that is historically situated in racism. I bring into our discussion Audre Lorde's idea that "Caring for myself is not self-indulgence, it is self-preservation, and that is an act of political warfare" (Lorde, 2017). Students begin to see how such indoctrination and mental unfreedom are useful in the perpetuation of oppression and destructive of *their own* humanity, as it is destructive to the humanity of others. Thus, they begin to see why their own mental freedom is essential for their own well-being and for creating a world that is just and free and compassionate. Here, they very naturally return to our conversations on *interbeing* and *Ubuntu*, as we explore the insight that our humanity depends on seeking radical freedom for ourselves and for others.

Our readings in *Radical Dharma* (williams, Owens, and Syedullah, 2016) offer us an intersectional expansion, as the authors explore their experiences of racism, sexism, homophobia, and more. As Rev. angel says:

> Radical Dharma is insurgence rooted in love, and all that love of self and others implies. It takes self-liberation to its necessary end by moving beyond personal transformation to transcend dominant social norms and deliver us into collective freedom.
>
> (williams, 2016, p. xi)

Radical love, compassion, and nurturing care means seeking this kind of radical freedom for ourselves and others. She tells us:

> Each community possesses, as Gandhi offered, a piece of the truth—of Dharma. When we seek the embodiment of these truths, giving ourselves permission to be more honest, more healed, more whole, more complete—when we become radical—neither the path of solely inward-looking liberation nor the pursuit of an externalized social liberation prevails; rather, a third space… emerges…. We cast our bodies into the third space that emerges when radically inhabiting the two: the inner and outer paths toward liberation.
>
> (williams, 2016, pp. xxi–xxii)

This third space that Rev. angel describes is the convergence toward which we've been aiming during the whole semester, and students recognize the connection to our previous texts right away. We discuss what the inner path toward liberation from racist indoctrination means for each of us and what the outer path toward liberation of our relationships, communities, and society means.

We lean on the invitation we find in *Radical Dharma* (williams, Owens, and Syedullah, 2016)—an invitation to get to work freeing ourselves so that we have the resources we need to build a more just world. I choose meditations led by Rev. angel and Lama Rod for these class sessions—meditations that talk us through sitting with the feelings that emerge as we reckon with our immersion in such violent systems. Spending time at the start of class by entering into the vulnerability of such emotion prepares us to engage in discussions that often feel risky or dangerous, especially in our current cultural climate. As we consider the powerful emotion that arises, we turn to the question of how we might take up anger, through Lama Rod Owens' book, *Love and Rage* (2020). As he explains:

> In my dharma training and in retreat, what I began to see was that my anger was valid, and that it was trying to teach me. In dharma communities where we're taught that we just need to suppress our anger and that anger is wrong… that's just another strategy that these spaces are using to control bodies, to police bodies. You know? Because our anger, especially if we're in dharma spaces, our anger is actually helping us to look at things that feel really off. I'm just not angry for the hell of it.
>
> (Owens, 2020, p. 36)

In class discussion, we connect Lama Rod's ideas back to Zenju Earthlyn Manuel's (2019) article and bell hooks' (2019) article. We watch talks Lama Rod has given where he explores grief and healing. He is one of the teachers doing some of the most *incredible work* on how we suffer so deeply, and remain bound and unfree, because we don't know what to do with our broken-heartedness. We compare and contrast this with the idea in *The Book of Joy* (Dalai Lama, Tutu, and Abrams, 2016) that anger is often self-defensive and motivated by our love for ourselves, even though it may prevent us from feeling and releasing our broken-heartedness into its full and free expression. The point of all of this is to consider what it means to have the freedom to *be*, to compassionately let ourselves *be as we are*, allowing *everything* that emerges. Lama Rod urges us to find space—to *breathe* space—wherein *we can be*, and feel, and nurture ourselves and others. In this space, we cultivate within ourselves the radical liberation and love that empowers us to act to make change in the world. Our final journal prompt engages students in reflection on precisely these questions and their own practice.

In our end-of-semester film, *Fierce Light: When Spirit Meets Action* (Ripper, 2008), we see examples of spiritual activism from around the world and across spiritual traditions and practices, insisting on radical justice. When we seek justice without radical love, the work can be exhausting and crushing, and we frequently neglect our tender human inner lives. When we seek love without radical liberation or radical justice, we stop short of the hard work of changing our world.

The Lessons and Surprises

I conclude these reflections with a glimpse of what this work has revealed and, really, reinforced for me, my own spiritual practice, and my work with students. I have always seen my students as more than simply their role as students in my course. I have always seen every one of them as a unique, irreplaceable, *full human being*, with struggles and triumphs, and suffering and joy, and pain and enthusiasm, and grief and hilarity. Going into this course, I hoped that they would find the connection between social justice action and their own inner liberation and well-being to be powerful and helpful in their lives. I did not anticipate that it would touch many of them as deeply as it did. As I engage with them in this course, their broken-heartedness, their yearning for relief and freedom, their yearning for love—from others and from themselves—and their growing understanding of the cages we impose on ourselves and others are all given voice, attention, and dialogic exploration. And because of our approach to the course, I can bring myself into the room in these ways, too—honest and vulnerable about the spiritual dimension of our lives. To some degree, most philosophical exploration engages these aspects of life, but it often does an intellectualized version of this work. This teaching experience has taught me to encourage a more liberated way of exploring these themes and questions—liberated because it allows in the emotional and the spiritual. I believe that these integrations, and this journeying together, bring to the classroom the kinds of exploration and dialogue that occur through spiritual direction.

Like all of us, of course, I find myself running, and preoccupied, and noisy inside, and sometimes tied up in knots. My own cages. Teaching this course reminds me to practice, myself. Thich Nhat Hanh says in writing (e.g., Hanh, 2001) and in an interview with Oprah,[10] that we can engage with other persons most beautifully with four Mantras: "Darling, I am here for you. Darling, I know you are there, and I am very happy. Darling, I know you suffer. Darling, I suffer. Please help me." This course reminds me to re-orient myself before I walk into the classroom—to be fully *here with them*—happy for their presence and present for the suffering we each might bring into the space. It reminds me to re-orient myself in this way both for *them* and *also for me*, so that I don't miss what I love about teaching because I'm distracted. I feel called to be a teacher, a witness, a learning partner, a guide. I can be a bit freer, a bit more deeply engaged, and honestly, a lot more joyful.

I have found myself whispering to myself as I head to class, "I'm just going to go in and love them for 90 minutes." Offering them my love means creating a space of compassion and care and openness and joy. This is openness and joy both within myself and within the classroom, making the classroom a space of *freedom to be*—in their full selves—to think and raise questions and offer critique, of course, and also a space *to feel*. It's a space where they can turn their attention to the small flame within that yearns for liberation and freedom. They can breathe air into that flame that deeply yearns for love—*radical* love for themselves and for others—and that yearns for *real community*. Together, we can fan that flame within each of us that can burn for real, radical collective liberation and justice, and be driven to *do something* about it. In their lives outside of our classroom, this will mean cultivating a practice themselves, and creating Sangha for themselves and others—including support from a therapist/counselor in their own mental health path. It will also mean speaking up for themselves and others, resisting domination in all the forms it takes, and working to create freedom, equity, and justice in the world.

Referring to what he learned from the Dalai Lama and Desmond Tutu, Douglas Abrams says:

> The more we make a different choice, to heal our own suffering, the more we can turn to others and help to address their suffering with the laughter-filled, tear-stained eyes of the heart. And the more we turn away from our self-regard to wipe the tears from the eyes of another, the more—incredibly—we are able to bear, to heal, and to transcend our own suffering. This was their true secret to joy.
>
> (Dalai Lama, Tutu, and Abrams, 2016, p. 305)

My own path of healing led me into this unique course space with students, and every time I teach it, I more easily remember to bring to them—and to all my students—the laughter-filled, tear-stained eyes of my own heart—to love, and to persist in the hard work of liberation and justice. I hope that our time together in this course can be a small part of students' own cultivation of a radical love and liberation, for themselves and for others, on the way to healing and justice.

Epilogue: Meditation Together

If I may, I would like to invite you to finish your reading of this chapter with a meditation.

Let us breathe together.

Please take a comfortable posture. Perhaps straighten your spine, if that works for you. Place your feet flat on the floor, or lie down, or shift your body in whatever way your body needs. Soften your gaze.

Maybe shrug your shoulders, gently move your head from side to side.

And take a deep breath. In through your nose and let it out through your mouth.

See if you can locate any tension in your body, or your mind. Maybe you find some tightness or anxiety, or maybe some sadness or anger.

Take a breath. See if you can breathe some space around this feeling you find. Loving breath. Exhale, releasing your grip on this feeling. Let it be. There's no need to hold it so tightly.

Once more. Inhale tender care and space for this feeling. Exhale and let it be present and free.

On your next in-breath, see the *you* who feels this feeling. Inhale love and compassion for yourself. Breathe in tenderness. Let the breath loosen the knots that grip you. Exhale to release and soften and create space for yourself to feel, and to be loved and to be free.

Once more. Inhale tender care and space for *you*. Exhale to let yourself be present and free and loved.

On your next in-breath, bring to mind others who suffer in our world, from harm or injustice or oppression. Inhale compassion and love for them. Breathe space within yourself for the emergence of a deep feeling of responsibility and a powerful, radical upsurge of care. Breathe oxygen into the loving fire of solidarity. Exhale to send love to all those who suffer or struggle or fight for liberation, and to nourish your fierce commitment to liberation and justice for all beings.

And one more. Inhale radical love, radical liberation, radical passion for justice. Exhale.

And now let us move out into the world with new clarity and power, resisting the violence and harm and indoctrination that wounds, and acting to create the just, equitable, loving world we have the power to create.

Notes

1 Reggie Hubbard gathered and nourished this unique community and created *Active Peace Yoga*, and I am deeply grateful to him, and thankful for his teaching, his work, and his friendship. He is now a sought-after teacher, speaker, and practitioner. Available at: www.activepeaceyoga.com

2 Further information about Plum Village can be found at their website.

3 According to Milan Rai in "Editorial: Working With, not For," in *Peace News*: For *Nonviolent* Revolution, "This quote is attributed to Lilla Watson, an indigenous Australian artist, activist and academic. It is said she used these words at the 1985 UN Decade for Women Conference in Nairobi, Kenya. Lilla Watson herself is not comfortable being credited as the sole author of these words. She feels that they came out of a collective process in an Aboriginal rights group that she was part of in the 1970s in Queensland, Australia." Rai, M. "Editorial: Working With, not For," Peace News: For Nonviolent Revolution. Available at: https://peacenews.info/node/9900/editorial-working-not.

4 While it is customary to refer to authors by their last name, I am opting to refer to Rev. angel Kyodo williams as Rev. angel because this is what is used in mindfulness practice and teaching communities.

5 We read several more articles from *True Peace Work* than I am able to include here.

6 The segment we watch is called "Taking Care of Anger." See: Hanh (2004).

7 Thay means "teacher," and we adopt this way of referring to Thich Nhat Hanh that is used in the Plum Village tradition.

8 A version of this 5-year-old child meditation can be found by following the link in the References. See: Hanh (2015).

9 It is essential to offer frequent reminders about privacy, vulnerability, and respecting and caring for each other both within our classroom space and outside of it.

10 This interview, "How to Listen with Compassion" is on Oprah Winfrey's "Super Soul Conversations" podcast. See: Hanh (2019d).

References

Biko, S. B. (2002). *I write what I like: Selected writings* (A. Stubbs, C.R., Editor). The University of Chicago Press. (Original work published 1978).

Dalai Lama. (2019a). Genuine compassion. In *True peace work: Essential writings on engaged Buddhism* (pp. 151–158). Parallax Press.
Dalai Lama. (2019b). Hope for the future: 1988. In *True peace work: Essential writings on engaged Buddhism* (pp. 341–347). Parallax Press.
Dalai Lama, Tutu, D., and Abrams, D. (2016). *The book of joy: Lasting happiness in a changing world.* Avery.
Engle, D. G. (director and writer). (2014). *Children of the light* [documentary film]. PeaceJam Foundation.
Fossella, T. (2011). Human Nature, Buddha Nature: An interview with John Welwood. *Tricycle: The Buddhist Review*, Spring.
Francis, M. J. and Pugh, M. (directors, writers, and producers), Francis, N., Kar, H., Moore, W., and Tan, C.-M. (producers). (2017). *Walk with me* [documentary film]. Speakit Films; SunnyMarch.
Freire, P. (1993). *Pedagogy of the oppressed* (M. B. Ramos, Trans.). Penguin Books. (Original work published 1970.)
Hanh, T. N. (1991). *Peace is every step: The path of mindfulness in everyday life.* Bantam Books.
Hanh, T. N. (2001). *Anger: Wisdom for cooling the flames.* Riverhead Books.
Hanh, T. N. (2004) *Taking care of anger. Excerpt from Ending the vicious circle of negative habits.* Plum Village. Available at: https://www.youtube.com/watch?v=9OvLOna5_1A
Hanh, T. N. (2015) Mindfulness of anger: embracing the child within. *On Being*. Available at: https://onbeing.org/blog/mindfulness-of-anger-embracing-the-child-within/
Hanh, T. N. (2019a). Community as a resource. In *True peace work: Essential writings on engaged Buddhism* (pp. 223–241). Parallax Press.
Hanh, T. N. (2019b). Suffering is not enough. In *True peace work: Essential writings on engaged Buddhism* (pp. 3–6). Parallax Press.
Hanh, T. N. (2019c). Why we need a global ethic. In *True peace work: Essential writings on engaged Buddhism* (pp. 295–302). Parallax Press.
Hanh, T. N. (2019d). Thich Nhat Hanh: How to listen with compassion. Interview by Oprah Winfrey. *Super Soul Conversations.* OWN Podcast. Available at: https://www.youtube.com/watch?v=Z3AtmPS1Wic
hooks, b. (2019). Toward a worldwide culture of love. In *True peace work: Essential writings on engaged Buddhism* (pp. 317–328). Parallax Press.
williams, a.K. (2016). *Introduction: Enter here: Radical challenge.* In a. Kyodo williams, L. R. Owens, and J. Syedullah, *Radical Dharma: Talking race, love, and liberation* (pp. xix–xxx). North Atlantic Books.
williams, a.K. (2017). It's Not All About Love Afterall. *TEDx Washington Square*, January 25. https://youtu.be/PztCw49OQ2g?feature=shared.
williams, a.K. (2019). Unlearning the Ways of the System [sermon]. *All Saints Church Padadena,* February 10. https://www.youtube.com/watch?v=lC-CxqTGxjk.
williams, a.K., Owens, L. R., and Syedullah, J. (2016). *Radical Dharma: Talking race, love, and liberation.* North Atlantic Books.
Lorde, A. (2017) *A burst of light: And other essays.* Ixia Press edition. Ixia Press, 2017.
Manuel, Z. E. (2019). Where the heart lives. In *True peace work: Essential writings on engaged Buddhism* (pp. 257–268). Parallax Press.
Owens, R. (2020). *Love and rage: The path of liberation through anger.* North Atlantic Books.

Ripper, V. (director and writer), Becker, M. and Spottiswood, G. (writers), Hawrysh, C. and Flahive, G. (producers). (2008). *Fierce light: When spirit meets action*. Fiercelight Films; National Film Board of Canada.
Sivaraksa, S. (2019). Buddhism in a world of change. In *True peace work: Essential writings on engaged Buddhism* (pp. 85–96). Parallax Press.
Stuparich, L. (director and producer). (2012). *Road to peace: Ancient Wisdom of the 14th Dalai Lama of Tibet*. Road to Peace Films.
Welwood, J. (1984). Principles of inner work: Psychological and spiritual. *The Journal of Transpersonal Psychology*, 16(1), 63–73.

Chapter 6

A Rhizomatic Reflection on Spiritual Direction, Embodiment, and Difference

Anthony Cruz Pantojas

Spirituality has been an essential part of humanity, influencing and shaping the way of life for centuries, and yet spirituality itself takes distinctly different forms for different cultures and eras. Over time, the desire to understand and experience this range of spiritualities has evolved into a diverse range of expressions, practices, and charisms that have moved beyond traditional religious identifiers in contexts like higher education, mental wellness, and healthcare settings. Today, as Pew Research reports steadily show, there is a growing number of people who identify as "nones": spiritual but not religious, spiritually seeking, questioning, and more (Smith, 2021). In a curation of the profiles of nones, AP News (Associated Press, 2023) reports that "there has been a dramatic increase in the number of people who are nonbelievers or unaffiliated with any organized religion… compris[ing] 30% or more of the adult population in the United States and Canada." This trend underscores diverse voices from around the globe and importantly clarifies the challenges, difficulties, and religious/philosophical negotiations undertaken by people who identify across the spectrum of secular, non-theist, and atheists. It has also impacted spiritual direction formation, popular culture, and academic discussions, leading to the need for a deeper engagement with historically underrepresented voices and scholarship in spiritual direction.

This chapter orients the importance of spiritual direction to those conditions that allow for the exploring, questioning, critiquing, and clarifying of values and sources in everyday life. Furthermore, this paper deploys the notion of the rhizome as a critical heuristic. I follow the theorizations of the rhizome from philosophers Gilles Deleuze, Félix Guattari, and Édouard Glissant, who engage in more dynamic and creative ways of experiencing the world. The rhizome comprises multiple points of departure and exit, diffractively offering possibilities to relate otherwise. This chapter is an invitation towards more capaciousness and consilience, creating more opportunities to engage with spirituality and accompaniment in renewed ways.

Afro-Caribbean Humanist Positionality

Positionality and spirituality are intrinsically intertwined, and through one's life journey, they can nurture one another. I hail from Borikén, more

DOI: 10.4324/9781003742852-6

commonly known as Puerto Rico. It was there in my homeland that I was exposed from a very young age to a multiplicity of religious, cultural, and spiritual practices that I did not fully understand. Yet, I honor that I was born into a social location that breathed and enculturated a triple consciousness. This polysemous being comes in part from being born in a colony of the United States in the Caribbean. At the same time, this complex reality allowed me to grow and I was exposed to Afro-based living traditions, Catholicism, Protestantism, Judaism, Islam, other spiritual orienting systems, and nontheist orientations. These cultural and wisdom traditions allude to im/migration of people and the tension between survival through syncretism, hybridization, and/or resistance for those continuously questioning and exploring their lives and the resources utilized for this work. Being moved to seriously consider my *lo cotidiano* [quotidian reality], I am called to invite faithful witnesses to the table to construct a world where collective flourishing is the ontological benchmark. Like Lefebvre (1988), the quotidian is a fecund site to explore what endures, what changes, and how relationships evolve. Witnessing *lo cotidiano* is also an important political activity to map and trace connections to power.

However, what this deeply reflected statement has not unpacked is the crucial role that creolization, migration, cuirness, and coloniality has played in the formation of my consciousness, lifestances, and spiritual and ethical practice. In other words, I am a proponent of quotidian experiences as sites of spirituality and new possibilities. This statement, however, also acknowledges that, in my own practice as an Afro-Caribbean Humanist/freethinker, educator, chaplain, and spiritual director, the colonial reality of my homeland played a fragmentary role in my life without my knowing it at the time. This moment served as an important consideration for me, and is echoed by Dr. Fernando Picó, who stated, "Todo el mundo quiere hablar y nadie quiere oír" [Everyone wants to talk and no one wants to hear] (Picó, 2014, p. 79). As a spiritual director of the global majority who hails from the Caribbean, this has multiple layers of meaning, understanding, and practice. Mainly, this phrase challenges the academically entrenched assumption that, for every word we hear, the response must be a well substantiated, articulated, and citable statement.

I carry within myself various traditions—Roman Catholicism, Judaism, Humanism, Afro-based spirituality, and others—that inform my bio-psycho-spiritual and social realities. I continuously hold, for example, being an Afro-Caribbean, cuir, neurodivergent, first-generation, low-income, and many other self-imposed labels. These are important to recognize, name, and center because they not only inform my life but also the ways in which I practice Spiritual Direction and relate across and beyond traditions, wisdom, and experiences that are leveraged in the process of radical accompaniment. The ways these come into a thread of relations can be synthesized by the words of Sephardic Rabbi Rifat Soncino who shares, "Spirituality cannot be imposed. It has to be discovered by each discerning individual" (Sonsino, 2002, p. 152).

Spiritual Direction and the Development of Liminal Space

Spirituality has always had a polyvalent nature and as such allows for a rich and meaningful liminal space that has been a refuge for those within the margins of religious, philosophical, and cultural traditions as well as those outside of them. It is through this understanding that the professionalization of "traditional" spaces provided by spiritual direction in the 21st century is beginning to be contested—there are now spaces where spiritual work and formation can be accessed that center queerness, the global majority, and wisdom beyond the Christian hegemony. Through these emerging new ways and spaces, spirituality becomes-yet-remains an important area for people from the global majority who seek to be in dialogue with their roots and (hi) stories, as well as deepening their meaning and purpose in their quotidian life in order to then accompany others in their own spiritual work. In the words of Caribbean scholar, M. Jacqui Alexander, the importance of relational work "through the Sacred becomes a way of embodying the remembering of self, if you will, a self that is neither habitually individuated nor unwittingly secularized" (Alexander, 2005, p. 298).

Spirituality is both a methodology and a practice that encompasses the human lived experience as a way of knowing and interpreting the inner and outer world by which we are surrounded. Similarly, such an approach can be applied to historical and cultural phenomena if there is a desire to unearth-and-reground the past and roots of a people.

The independent writer and philosopher Pedro Lebrón Ortiz provides an alternative space from an intellectual approach to those in the Caribbean. Ortiz speaks about the concept of *cimarronaje analéctico* defined as "una manera de encarnar la libertad a través de la huida ontología del mundo de la euromodernidad en función de la afirmación de un mundo propio, utilizando la memoria y filosofía ancestral como coordenadas" [a way of embodying freedom through the ontological flight from the world of Euromodernity in function of the affirmation of a world of one's own, using ancestral memory and philosophy as coordinates] (Ortiz, 2020, p. 37). The concept of *cimarronaje analéctico* uplifts the historical, cultural, and lived experiences of the Afro Caribbean and how the processes of self-denial, oppression, and negation occur in the mind. At the same time, the concept recognizes where the Afro-diasporic and Afro-indigenous bodies have been and decides to act in ways of resistance to the colonial, neoliberal, and Western frameworks. Thus, spiritual direction can be practiced in this same understanding, sensibility, and orientation.

The field and practice of spiritual direction offers the ostensive aim of being objective/totally differentiated at times, and yet this is not what certain communities need—though, undeniably, there must be set boundaries, practitioner ethics, and confidentiality in place. Furthermore, the growing number of nones, spiritual but not religious, spiritually fluid, and those with multiple religious or philosophical belongings need spaces where they can just *be*. In a personal and simplistic way, I define my Caribbean spiritual direction practice as a form of spiritual work of accompaniment with parallaxic possibilities. Spirituality is an epistemological structure and methodology that acknowledges intentional ways to think of interstices of culture, identity, and of *being* differently. It is accessible and intervenes in the everyday as a force we all create and in which we participate. This interdependence and acknowledgement lead to collective flourishing.

After establishing this foundation for both spirituality and spiritual direction, I will expand on some of the threads that emerged from the intersections between spirituality, education, and spiritual direction. Thus, I must bring as interlocutors those who can, from a contemporary lens, analyze dynamics of power, community organizing, and education. Moreover, by utilizing these scholars one can gauge the importance of spirituality in the formation of the human. As decolonial educational scholars Wane, Todorova, and Todd (2019) state:

> Although education is accessible to more people than ever before in human history, the dominant paradigm focuses solely on knowledge, skill, and material acquisition that neglects the meaning and purpose of life. This creates a huge void in learners and produces a huge number of people who are unhappy, unfulfilled, restless, lost, or desperate.
>
> (p. 3)

This quote in the context of spiritual direction addresses that there are opportunities for both proximality and intimacy. In this way education, knowledge, and experiences also take into consideration and equally validate the existential dimension of the human condition and the unfolding life in its messiness and complexity. Thus, through the art and practice of spiritual direction, these dimensions might glean possibilities for meaning-making and holistic life integration leading towards a recasting of purpose and vocation(s).

Spiritual Direction and Reflexive Meaning-Making

One of the resources at the disposal of a spiritual director is the verbatim, a practice shared with other professional fields like chaplaincy. Though it tends to be predominantly used during the period of clinical psycho-spiritual education (CPE) training, it remains an essential method to critically explore intrapersonal, interpersonal, and intrapsychic dimensions. In addition, spiritual directors are required to be in a mentoring relationship with a more seasoned director to promote accountability and to ensure system analyses are sharpened and that growing edges, biases, prejudices, or unethical behavior are kept in a mode of checks and balances. One of the techniques that I utilize during my spiritual direction is listening for the expansiveness of the directee and their community of origin or chosen community.

In this brief vignette, I share a spiritual direction encounter that took place a few months after having completed my spiritual direction training at Still Harbor in 2021. As an Afro-Caribbean spiritual director, I have made a commitment to take seriously the work of the self—or perhaps our multiple selves—and the wisdom that emerges from lived experience as a valid source of knowledge, as well as my positionality as a cuir and diasporic subject.

The directee in this vignette voiced one of the reasons why they wanted to be accompanied by me through the following statement:

> I've been waiting to find a spiritual director with a more common background, one that understands how to navigate my spiritual traditions. I already have a therapist, and I recognize the distinctions in roles. This is where I am at.

When my directee made the initial declaration, I was actually troubled and curious with the statement. Their presumption of a shared background made me wary about being positioned stereotypically as "the one" for them, meaning a mythic and marginalized identity to be commodified by persons and institutions for consumption (Peña, 2022). Through parallel processing, I reflect on the misconception that there is only one and instead respond by working towards relating to and being in solidarity with those not historically visible and co-create new spaces in the field of spiritual direction. Like many other encounters, there is indeed a need for trained spiritual directors from the global majority who are also dedicated to healing, care, liberation, and freedom.

At this point in time, I do not know of any empirical study that has been done surveying spiritual directors of color. There are only a handful of trained spiritual directors who hail from the global majority that openly identify as humanists or nontheists, as well as cuir, and who have developed an embodied transcultural and transreligious way of life.

As I reflect again on these words, I continue to ruminate on the lack of understanding or interest in the practice of spiritual direction for those who identify as nontheists, nones, and spiritual but not religious. As my directee perceived, spiritual directors are not psychologists, mental health counselors, or therapists. In my practice for example, I view my work as facilitating, reflecting, and weaving together words, images, musings, and creations that illuminate the inner worlds that are emerging or becoming known during our encounters. And yet, I do want to point out the growing recognition of the role that spirituality plays as part of a holistic model of wellbeing and mental health—for example, a combination of graduate-level theological training, clinical psycho-spiritual education, and spiritual direction.

We must recognize the historical and everyday reality of moments of silence, erasure, negation, and marginalization that are experiences very much present and embodied in the lives of people from the global majority and those with transgressing identities. In the words of Lucumí priest and professor Carlos Decena:

> It claims a knowing, a conocimiento, that recognizes our whole bodies as instruments for an expanded apprehension of the world(s). This opaque wisdom of the ancestras, and transcestras, the joining of the street, body-mind cunning of those walking the edges of what can be known.
>
> (Decena, 2023, p. 57)

The quotation is applicable to spiritual direction in several ways. First, it recognizes that we inherently have a sense or capacity of knowing that guides our lives and ways of existing, that our lives can be whole or in process; it also illuminates how our bodies, through the quotidian, are informed by context, and that lived experiences develop a form of not just surviving, but flourishing that can be known to some and yet unknown to others. Furthermore, it validates how there is a multiplicity of wisdom in everyday life that catalyzes us into a fierce exploration of how navigating multiple worlds is both already accessible and an invitation into possibilities in the here and now.

Spiritual Direction as Care and Liberation

Care is integral to spiritual direction, accompaniment, and resilience building. Through the processes of racial capitalism/white supremacy, we have been taught to unlearn the content and character of care. Without a doubt, "care," in the hegemonic grind, can be rendered trite or a lifeless policy. However, when many of us are "living through" states of dispossession and death, embodied and truly present care is so important to recognize. Care is extended to me through the generosity of ideas, of allowing myself to breathe, and inviting an uninhibited me. I constantly think about the character of the care we give and receive.

The history of spiritual direction impacts how we organize and resist. Movements towards collective liberation need not just offer respite, but support spaces to be, to be tended to in order to sustain this important work. I have experienced burnout, "equity fatigue" in primarily white spaces, and generally in the work that I do with others. I feel compelled to "do it all," which inevitably leads me to not being present in the work that I find important. I often have to step back when I'm overwhelmed and collect all the thoughts I have that are contributing to burnout or my being overwhelmed. Slowing down is still difficult for me, but I'm getting better. When burnout occurs, people have been encouraged to rest, and to appraise what needs they have that must be met. I think being clear with ourselves, and the groups to whom we are accountable to, about the various needs we have, helps to mobilize wellbeing and freedom for all.

When thinking about my personal praxis in spiritual direction, I am invited to think through mutuality, accountability, and conflict in more rigorous ways. I draw inspiration from adrienne maree brown where she states, "Resilience is unveiled when we are triggered, injured, heartbroken, attacked, challenged. I am curious about our general resilience as social justice actors in a traumatizing world, and as collectives of people shaping the next phase of human evolution" (brown, 2018, p. 126). When we tend to the root of injustice, we are much more able to come up with more spaciousness in terms of responding to it. I think about brown's gesturing to transformative justice that creates a more reparative mode of harm and trauma. We bear witness to each other's humanness and come together to be in the right relationship.

I am conceptualizing the ways in which to instantiate more sustainable practices and relationships. The multivalent ways in which spiritual direction can be enacted is refreshing. I appreciate the candor and vulnerability others in this volume present their work and experiences. Spiritual direction speaks to me in the sense of addressing the whole person and providing that same contextualization to groups, organizations, and even social movements. Spiritual direction is needed in a time where we are reckoning with states of debility and death. Our spiritual needs must be addressed in order for movements to be sustained.

Epilogue

I offer a reflection on the poem "To These Poets for Tato Laviera" by Sandra María Esteves. The poem serves as a window into the Afro-diasporic imagination and traces coordinates of lineages, memory, and the transgression of spatial and temporal limits. This imagination plumbs the depths of collective wisdom to instantiate the otherwise that both reclaims and invites us to awaken our senses and capacity for repair, liberation, and freedom. These crossings are not made alone but actualized *en comunidad encarnada y mística*. They come through the bodies and voices of the historical present through words that are simultaneously disruptive and caresses, through the spiritual direction sessions we hold, we offer, the ceremonies and rituals we tend.

The contemporary practice of spiritual direction becomes an act of ancestral fidelity. We are receiving transmission. The ancestors who knew how to hold paradox without collapsing it into false resolve. The elder who understood that repairs happen not through individual enlightenment alone but through the collective work of imagination; whose "verses that lift us from the abyss" modeled for us what it means to be custodians of wisdom that "circulates in the river of our being" (Esteves, 2010, p. 3).

This is the work carried forward. To let the old pathways inform the new. To recognize that when we practice spiritual direction with another navigating their cultural identity, we are not separate from the Bomba dancer whose body remembers what colonization tried to erase. We are not distant from the initiate who bends towards the mysteries with the same reverence our ancestors bent toward survival and sovereignty. The tools they left us—the words, the rhythms, the rituals of return: these are not decorative or hallowed. They are epistemological. They teach us to know, how to imagine, how to repair.

To close this chapter is not to finish the work. It is to acknowledge that we do not journey alone. That every word spoken and entrusted in spiritual direction, every ritual tended, every door opened to welcome the forgotten and the marginalized, every bridge built across difference—these echoes of ancestral whispers are urgent with the task of liberation. We are contemporary raconteurs of our own becoming. And in the company of those who came before and those who will come after, we continue the crossing: toward freedom, toward repair, and toward the shores of creation where all our names are finally spoken in the language of home; and "con bendiciones recibidos [sic] en muchísimo aché" (Esteves, 2010, p. 119).

References

Alexander. M. J. (2005). *Pedagogies of crossing: meditations on feminism, sexual politics, memory, and the sacred.* Duke University Press.

Associated Press. (2023). The nones. *AP Projects.* Available at: https://projects.apnews.com/features/2023/the-nones/index.html

Brown, A. M. (2017). *Emergent strategy: Shaping change, changing worlds.* AK Press.

Castillo-Garsow, M. (Ed.). (2017). *¡Manteca!: An anthology of Afro-Latin@ poets.* Arte Público Press.

Decena, C. U. (2023). *Circuits of the sacred: A faggotology in the Black Latinx Caribbean.* Duke University Press.

Esteves, S. M. (2010). To these poets: For Tato Laviera. *Sandra María Esteves.* Available at: https://www.sandraesteves.com/images/ToThesePoets.2010.pdf

Levebvre, M. (1988). *They have uncrowned him: From liberalism to apostasy—the conciliar tragedy.* Angelus Press.

Ortiz, P. L. (2020). *Filosofía del cimarronaje.* Editora Educación Emergente.

Peña, L. G. (2022). *Community as rebellion: A syllabus for surviving academia as a woman of color.* Haymarket Books.

Picó, F. (2014). *Vocaciones caribeñas* (Segunda edición). Ediciones Callejón.

Smith, G. A. (2021). About three-in-ten U.S. adults are now religiously unaffiliated. *Pew Research Center's Religion and Public Life Project*, December 14. https://www.pewresearch.org/religion/2021/12/14/about-three-in-ten-u-s-adults-are-now-religiously-unaffiliated/

Sonsino, R. (2002). *Six Jewish spiritual paths: A rationalist looks at spirituality.* Jewish Lights Publishing.

Spiritual directee. (2021). Personal interview.

Wane, N. N., Todorova, M. S., and Todd, K. L. (Eds.). (2019). *Decolonizing the spirit in education and beyond: Resistance and solidarity.* Springer Nature.

Chapter 7

Kenotic Mysticism, Social Identity, and Leadership Formation in the Spiritual Direction of Clare of Assisi

Corné J. Bekker

The 13th-century Christian figure, Clare of Assisi (1193/4–1253 C.E.), was the first woman to construct a religious rule of life in Christianity. The organization she founded, the Poor Clares—as the Order of Saint Clare is often referred to, as well as the Second Order of Saint Francis—continues to flourish and serve the world more than 800 years later (Gregg, 2018). This chapter explores the spiritual direction model employed by Clare, specifically as found in her letters to Agnes of Prague (1211–1282 C.E.). Agnes was a Bohemian princess who opted for a life of radical poverty and service to the poor, influenced by the preaching and theology of the mendicant Franciscan friars in her country. Grounded in socio-rhetorical criticism, a repetitive-progressive pattern analysis of Clare's letters to Agnes locates Clare within the domain of a servant leader, providing transformative spiritual direction to her followers. As this chapter strives to show, Clare's servant leadership is fueled by kenotic mysticism.[1] Seen through the lens of social identity theory, Clare roots her ministry and direction offered to Agnes in her "ardent desire for the Poor Crucified" (1Lag13).[2] Kenotic mysticism and servant leadership are closely linked in Clare's writings in an interdependent dynamic system of personal and communal transformation through radical self-emptying fueled by a commitment to Jesus Christ. Kenotic mysticism allows the leader to transcend narrow selfhood and facilitates a radical commitment to others in service. The spiritual direction of Clare of Assisi offers spiritual directors a model and approach to serving those they direct through compassionate servant leadership and kenotic mutuality.

Historical Contexts of Clare of Assisi and Agnes of Prague

Clare of Assisi was the first Christian female leader to write a religious rule sanctioned by pontifical approval (Carney, 1993, p. 19). Imbued with the evangelical vision she received from the preaching of Francis of Assisi (1182–1226 C.E.), she rejected the prestige and privileges that her aristocratic family offered and instead opted for a life of religious service and in doing so constructed a new kind of monastic life which is described by

DOI: 10.4324/9781003742852-7

Karecki and Wroblewski (2003a, p. 3) as, "an enclosed contemplative life in an urban setting with highest poverty." The enclosed community of sisters that Clare founded at San Damiano, Assisi, was characterized, amongst other attributes, by:

(a) a contemplative focus on Christ (Karecki and Wroblewski, 2000b, p. 17);
(b) the primacy of the Bible as the Word of God (Karecki and Wroblewski, 2000c, p. 13);
(c) a counter-cultural ideology (Karecki and Wroblewski, 2001, p. 15);
(d) a preferential option for the poor (Bartoli, 1993, p. 7);
(e) an appreciation for mission (Karecki and Wroblewski, 2001, p. 13);
(f) charismatic healings (Duw, 1992, p. 14);
(g) and (g) service to others (Karecki and Wroblewski, 2001, p. 10).

The religious community that Clare started quickly spread around the rest of Italy, Europe, and the world.

Agnes of Prague was the daughter of King Přemysl Ottokar I and Queen Constance of Bohemia (Karecki and Wroblewski, 2003a, p. 6). Several high-level suitors were proposed for Agnes at a young age—Henry VII of Germany and Henry III of England were two. Agnes was finally betrothed to Frederick II, Holy Roman Emperor (1194–1250 C.E.) (Mueller, 2003, p. xvii). Influenced by the preaching of the missionary brothers of Francis, whom she heard preaching in 1232 (Armstrong and Brady, 1982, p. 189), she rejected the alliance (De Robeck, 1954, p. 55). Instead, she used her royal dowry to build a hospital, a monastery for women, and a small convent for friars supporting the sisters (Mueller, 2003, p. xviii). Agnes herself joined the monastery she built and requested sisters who followed the form of life of Clare's community in San Damiano (Mueller, 2003, p. xviii). Agnes supported Clare in her pursuit of contemplative poverty and sought the same privilege of poverty from Pope Gregory IX (1145–1241 C.E.) that Clare received (Karecki and Wroblewski, 2003a, p. 11). Clare wrote four letters to Agnes to guide and lead her in her commitment to the Franciscan ideal and Christ (Armstrong and Brady, 1982, pp. 189–206). These letters were lost to modern scholars until 1915 when Walter Seton discovered them in a 14th-century manuscript (Karecki and Wroblewski, 2003b, p. 5). Repetitive-progressive texture analysis of the letters to Agnes of Prague opens new avenues in reading these texts. It provides contemporary readers and scholars with an opportunity to explore the leadership and spirituality of Clare of Assisi further.

The Kenotic Mysticism and Servant Leadership of Clare of Assisi

Clare's writings are rich in theology and spirituality. Recent scholarship has noted her theological leadership in the formative years of the Franciscans and as an original interpreter of Scripture (Pryds, 2012, p. 136). Her leadership has been described as authentic (Gerundt and Warode, 2018, p. 1), follower-focused (Freeman, 2019, p. 28), transformational (Gregg, 2018, p. 49), and as indicative of servant leadership (Bekker, 2013, p. 17). Her theology, deeply rooted in Christian Scriptures and the Christ-centered vision of Francis, is fueled by a desire to know her Lord in the mutuality of his suffering and poverty. In light of the constraints of this chapter, the focus is firmly placed on Clare's kenotic mysticism and leadership dynamics, as found in the letters to Agnes of Prague. Greenleaf's (1998, pp. 18–19) seminal work on servant leadership defines the concept as follows:

> The servant-leader is servant first… It begins with the natural feeling that one wants to serve, to serve first. The conscious choice brings one to aspire to lead. He or she is sharply different from the person who is leader first, perhaps because of the need to assuage an unusual power drive or to acquire material possessions.

Clare's absolute commitment to poverty, her refusal to accept the markings and privileges of the religious temporal powers of her time, and her vocation of service place her within the domain of a servant leader. Patterson (2003, p. 2), building on Greenleaf's definition, describes servant leadership as a virtuous theory comprising seven virtuous constructs. These virtues are:

(a) love,
(b) humility,
(c) altruism,
(d) vision,
(e) trust,
(f) empowerment,
and (g) service.

Successive repetitive-progressive texture analysis of Clare's letters to Agnes identifies these virtues as integral to her vision and ideology.

The spirituality of Clare of Assisi falls within the domain of Christian mysticism. Ledoux (1997, p. 27) defines Christian mysticism as "the experience of the interior and unifying encounter with the Divine Infinite that is the foundation of the Divine Being and of all existence." Clare's mysticism has been described as:

(a) profoundly Christological (Kourie, 1993, p.125);
(b) affectionate (Mueller, 2003, p. 103);
(c) Scriptural (Kourie, 1993, p. 126):
(d) theological (Ledoux, 1997, p. 25);
(e) incarnational (Kourie, 1993, p. 125);
and (f) kenotic (Karecki, 2000b, p. 2).

Clare's practice of voluntary poverty is rooted in the desire to imitate the *kenosis* [self-emptying] of Christ (Teresa, 1995, p. 109) as expressed within the Christological hymn of *Philippians* 2:5–11 (Kourie, 1993, p. 126). The *Philippians* hymn has been described as a stance of mimetic Christological leadership in the early Church in stark contrast to the timocratic leadership preferences of the Roman Empire (Bekker, 2021, p. 1). Francis and Clare's theological ideal of mimetic reenactment of the kenosis of Christ is what fueled their understanding of conversion and transformation (Bekker and Buchard, 2015, p. 3). Kenosis in Franciscan theology (Cronin, 1992, p. 1) is seen as a "resolute divesting of the person of every claim of self-interest so as to be ready to live the Gospel of Christ in every aspect of living, freed from the dictates of personal preference." Clare's voluntary divesting of power, prestige, and possessions finds its theological context in her deep desire to follow in the footsteps of the kenotic Christ who emptied Himself and embraced poverty for the sake of others. Kourie (1993, p. 124) describes Clare's commitment to radical poverty as transformational: "Clare's practice of poverty had as its aim the radical transformation of the person, the abolition of a narrow selfhood and the silencing of the all too natural tendency toward fragmentation and purely functional consciousness." The kenotic mysticism of Clare leads to human authentication (Kourie, 1993, p. 125) that allows the leader to enter the world of followers and focus on their humanity in the pursuit of service.

Socio-rhetorical Criticism and the Letters of Clare to Agnes of Prague

The letters of Clare to Agnes of Prague are of primary value in reconstructing the leadership approach and spiritual direction of Clare of Assisi. These letters have "high research value" (Cai, 2022, p. 3) and have received renewed attention from scholars interested in exploring the contribution of Clare to theology spirituality, and spiritual direction (Mooney, 2016). The use of repetitive-progressive pattern analysis of these letters holds significant promise in uncovering the broad theological and spiritual themes contained in them. Repetitive-progressive pattern analysis is part of a more extensive approach to interpreting texts known as socio-rhetorical criticism. Robbins (1996a, p. 1) proposes a multi-dimensional approach to the analysis of texts and named this methodological stance socio-rhetorical criticism. Robbins writes:

> rather than being another method for interpreting texts, socio-rhetorical interpretation is an interpretive, analytical approach that evaluates and reorients its strategies as it engages in multi-faceted dialogue with the texts and other phenomena within its purview. The approach does not claim to be comprehensive. Rather, the claim is that the approach uses

> the insights of sociolinguistics, semiotics, and ethnography in an interactionist philosophical mode that sets ancient, modern, and post-modern systems of thought in energetic dialogue with one another.
>
> (Robbins, 1996a, p. 1)

Robbins (1996a) attempts to integrate all the recent developments in linguistic, social, and cultural studies in a highly programmed methodology that has as its purpose to not only enlarge our understanding of the social and cultural dimensions of the text but also to facilitate new avenues of exploration in textual interpretation such as organizational leadership. It is important to note that as much as socio-rhetorical criticism is a new approach to text analysis, it is based on and incorporates the accomplishments of past scholars working in varied fields, ranging from textual analysis, linguistic studies, sociology, anthropology, and cultural observations (Gowler, 1994, p. 1). This new integrated approach to textual analysis introduces an inevitable paradigm shift in how one perceives, understands, and uses texts. Instead of seeing a text as a mere window through which one perceives meaning, one now focuses on the several layers or textures within the text as the key to interpretation. Robbins (1996a, p. 1) writes:

> guided by the metaphor of a text as a tapestry rather than a site of windows and mirrors, socio-rhetorical interpretation has begun to focus not only on multiple textures of a text but also on multiple discourses that interweave with one another within those textures. The interweaving of multiple textures and discourses within a text creates an environment in which signification, meanings, and meaning effects interact with one another in ways that no one method can display. Only an approach that is highly programmatic, complexly variegated, and readily adaptable can begin to engage and exhibit the rich world that texts bring into the life of humans as they live, work, struggle, suffer, die, celebrate, and commemorate together.

Socio-rhetorical analysis of ancient texts has not only opened a variety of new avenues for the textual, social, and cultural analysis of texts, but it has also provided us with a new context for multi-disciplinary exchange and discussion on the meaning, effect, and use of texts (Gowler, 1994, p. 12). This widening of rhetorical inquiry has also been extended to the writings of Francis of Assisi (Bekker and Buchard, 2015) as well as to Clare's letters to Agnes of Prague (Bekker, 2013). To structure his integrated approach to socio-rhetorical analysis of texts, Robbins (1996a, 1996b) proposes five broad categories of investigation:

- The **inner texture** of the text explores the text's inner textual texture;
- The **intertexture** of the text, which explores the intertextual texture of text;

- The text's **social and cultural texture** explores the social and cultural dimensions;
- The **ideological texture** of the text explores the ideological inner dynamics of the text;
- The **sacred texture** of the text.

Socio-rhetorical analysis is not a static approach to textual analysis but is constantly developing and exploring further-integrated social, cultural, linguistic, and rhetorical avenues for interpretation. The discussion now turns to the subset of inner texture analysis within the domain of socio-rhetorical criticism, namely repetitive-progressive texture – this is the approach that forms the methodological approach in this chapter in exploring the kenotic mysticism, social identity, and leadership formation in the spiritual direction of Clare of Assisi to Agnes of Prague.

Repetitive-Progressive Texture in Texts

The four letters of Clare to Agnes are typical of 13th-century letter writing in structure and are "rhetorically and metaphorically expressive" (Cai, 2022, p. 2). The letters contain numerous and repetitive use of "symbolism and metaphors" (Cai, 2022, p. 2) that reveal Clare's theological framework for her leadership and the spiritual direction she offers to Agnes. The use of repetitive-progressive analysis to explore these medieval letters serves to identify and analyze the underlying conceptual framework in Clare's communication and direction. Repetitive-progressive texture analysis forms part of the "inner texture" analysis in Robbins' (1996a, 1999b) schema. Reading a text is a complex process (De Beaugrande and Dressler, 1981) in which the text becomes "part of a communication transaction" (Vorster, 1989, p. 22). This "communication transaction" should be of great importance for readers of ancient manuscripts. Great attention should be given to how we bridge the gap of hundreds of years when we read these texts. We must ask how much of the meaning that we find in these texts comes from the original author, reflecting the original setting, and how much of the meaning derived do we bring to the text?

According to Robbins (1996a, pp. 27–28), the act of reading is the beginning of the exploration of the "inner texture" of the text. In the act of reading, the worlds of the author—real and implied—and reader—real and implied—combine to form this communication transaction. Robbins' socio-rhetorical analysis uses the text's inner texture to explore the interaction between the author, the text, and the reader (Robbins, 1996a, p. 30). To illustrate where this method of inner texture fits into the communication process, Robbins (1996a, p. 29) modifies the diagrams of Chatman (1978, p. 151) and Rimmon-Kenan (1983, p. 86) to include his method of unlocking the signs of meaning given by the author in the text (see Table 7.1 below).

Table 7.1 The Inner Texture of the Text

Real author	Implied author	→	**Inner texture**	→	Narrator & characters	→	→	→	Implied reader	Real reader/ audience

The rhetorical axis of communication →

In Robbins's modified diagram (see Table 7.1), the inner texture appears amongst the axis of the implied author, the narrator, and the characters, who function as the communication vehicles of the message. In the past, at this interpretation stage, the reader would focus on formulating a profile of the real author and audience that stood outside the text. Language and text structure would not feature as the central area of focus. Socio-rhetorical analysis aims to return to the reader, identify or explore the text's inner texture, and isolate the main areas of interest or intent of communication of the real/implied author and the real/implied reader or audience. It then takes this approach to the text even further and includes two further insights (Robbins, 1996a, p. 30):

> The results of this scholarly investigation into the identity and nature of the real/implied author and the real/implied reader or audience are brought into dialogue with other academic investigations of the text. Thus, a more holistic picture is presented of the possible meanings of the text.

The second important insight that Robbins' inner texture brings to the table of textual interpretation is the consent that the real reader or audience is an integral part of the construction of the inner text. Borrowing heavily from the insights of Anglo-American new criticism, Russian formalism, and French structuralism, Robbins (1996a, p. 30) reminds us that "a text does not truly become a text until someone reads it." For Robbins (1996a, p. 30), it is clear that readers are as much involved with the communication of meaning as the author. Robbins (1996a, p. 30) states: "As soon as readers do this [reading], however, their world of meanings and meaning effects works interactively with meanings and meaning effects from the ancient Mediterranean world to create the meaning and meaning effects of the text." According to Robbins (1996a, 1996b), the arena of inner texture is, in essence, the assimilation of various interpretative techniques drawn from a wide variety of sources with the intent to present a more holistic picture of the texture of the text. In this assimilation, this method's apparent strengths and weaknesses are found. Hopefully, this approach will unlock greater meaning in the text, taking the interaction between the real/implied author and the implied/real readers seriously. This focus on the interaction between author and audience in this methodological approach is helpful in the quest to further identify and analyze the leadership relationship and direction offered by Clare to Agnes in the four letters.

Robbins (1996a, 1996b) identifies five areas of exploration in the study of the inner texture of the text:

- **Repetitive-progressive texture;**
- **Opening-middle-closing texture;**
- **Narrational texture;**
- **Argumentative texture;**
- **Sensory aesthetic texture.**

Robbins (1996a, pp. 46–50) formulates his repetitive-progressive texture of the text based on the work of Tannehill (1975, 1989) on Luke/Acts, Trible's (1978, 1984) literary-feminist approach to Biblical narratives, and Alter's (1981) treatise on the nature of Biblical narratives. Armed with Tannehill's and Alter's insights and heavily influenced by the work of Neirynck (1972) on duality and tripartite expressions in the Gospel of Mark, Robbins (1981, 1982, 1984, 1987) published numerous articles and a book, mainly on the Gospel of Mark, that merged all of these rhetorical devices into a singular workable approach to determine the repetitive-progressive structure of the text. More recently, Robbins (1994a, 1994b, 1994c, 1994d, 1996a, p. 48) has been influenced by the work of Scott and Dean (1993) using word diagrams to determine a "sound map" of the Sermon on the Mount in Matthew's Gospel. Robbins (1996a, pp. 48–49) describes this subsequent development in the quest for the repetitive-progressive structure of the text:

> At this stage, the interpreter assigns only basic lexical meanings to the words in the text. This procedure withholds fuller meanings to allow sign and sound patterns to emerge. In other words, the emphasis is on the relations of the signs and sounds rather than the content and the meanings. At this stage, the interpreter is exploring primary process and form, a structured movement that produces meaning process and meaning effect.

For Robbins (1996a, p. 49), this synthesized approach to the determination of the repetitive-progressive texture holds the promise of a new window into the meaning of the text. It is a determined effort to take repetition and progression seriously in the quest for the meaning of a given text. Robbins (1996a, p. 50) proposes five possible questions in the rhetorical analysis of the repetitive-progressive texture of the text:

- What patterns emerge from the repetition of specific topics in the text?
- What topics replace other topics in the progression of the text?
- Is there continual repetition of the same word throughout the unit, or is there slight modification at almost every progressive stage?
- Does the progression bring certain kinds of words together but not others?
- Is there repetition in steps that creates a context for a new word progression?

To illustrate the particular repetitive-progressive structure of a specific text, it is helpful to make lists of words or phrases that repeatedly appear in the unit in the same or a modified form (Robbins 1996b, p. 8). The next section of this chapter presents several repetitive-progressive patterns in the letters of Clare of Assisi to Agnes of Prague using Patterson's (2003) theory of servant leadership. These are used to explore Clare's spirituality and leadership in a quest to describe her approach to spiritual direction.

Servant Leadership in the Letters of Clare of Assisi to Agnes of Prague

Patterson (2003, p. 2) proposes a theoretical model of servant leadership where the concept is defined as a virtuous theory comprising seven virtuous constructs:

(a) agapáo love,
(b) humility,
(c) altruism,
(d) vision,
(e) trust,
(f) empowerment,
and (g) service.

These seven virtues are used as a matrix to explore possible repetitive-progressive patterns in Clare's letters to Agnes. The repetitive progressive patterns that emerge in the text are used to analyze the spirituality and leadership of Clare of Assisi. Patterson (2003, p. 3) makes use of Winston's (2002, p. 5) definition of agapáo love as moral love, "doing the right thing at the right time and for the right reasons." Patterson (2003, p. 3) further describes this "love" as having esteem for followers, honoring them, and having their best interest at heart.

Agnes never met Clare (Mueller, 2003, p. 8), so it is astonishing that she still chose to associate herself with Clare and her order at its beginning stages. It was not as highly organized as the Benedictine order right next to her family's castle. Clare's objective in writing to Agnes can be summed up at the end of her salutations in the first letter (1Lag34): "that by their help we may merit the mercy of Jesus Christ, and together with You may merit to enjoy the everlasting vision." Clare's love for and commitment to Agnes is not based on social relationship but, as cited above, on their mutual "desire for the Poor Crucified" (line 13, p. 191) and is communicated in her letters as she desires to teach Agnes to embrace this path of joy (Mueller, 2003, p. 9). The letters to Agnes are acts of selfless love intended to lead Agnes to true fulfillment and joy.

When Clare's references to Agnes in her letters are analyzed, clear repetitive-progressive patterns of honor, esteem, and care emerge (see Table 7.2).

Table 7.2 Repetitive-progressive pattern illustrating Clare's references to Agnes.

First Letter		*Second Letter*		*Third Letter*		*Fourth Letter*	
1LAg1	esteemed and most holy virgin Lady Agnes daughter of the most excellent and illustrious King of Bohemia	2LAg1	daughter of the King of kings handmaid of the Lord of lords, most worthy spouse of Jesus Christ very distinguished queen Lady Agnes	3LAg1	Agnes most venerable lady sister in Christ blood-sister of the illustrious king of Bohemia sister and spouse of the most high King of the heavens	4LAg1	illustrious queen spouse of the Lamb of the eternal King Lady Agnes special daughter
1LAg8	virgin	2LAg4	diligent imitator of the Father	3LAg10	dearest	4LAg3	Agnes
1LAg12	most beloved sister Lady worthy of great respect spouse and the mother and the sister of my Lord Jesus Christ	2LAg7	an imitator of the holiest poverty	3LAg11	O Lady most beloved in Christ joy of the angels crown of your sisters	4LAg4	mother and daughter spouse of the King
1LAg24	a sister, spouse, and mother of the Son of the Father of the Most High and of the glorious Virgin	2LAg18	poor virgin	3LAg40	dearest one	4LAg7	spouse of Christ
1LAg31	Your Excellency Your holiness	2LAg20	most noble queen			4LAg15	O queen spouse of Jesus Christ
		2LAg24	dearest sister and lady			4LAg17	Dearest daughter spouse of the most high King
						4LAg27O	queen of the heavenly King
						4LAg36	blessed daughter
						4LAg39	dearest daughter

When these repetitive patterns in the letters are listed next to one another, a fuller picture of the conceptual and theological framework of Clare's leadership and direction approach emerges. It is worthwhile to consider both the repetitious and progressive patterns that are highlighted in these texts in order arrive at a richer analysis.

Clare addresses Agnes with terms of:

(a) **honor**: *Lady* (3LAg11), *Lady Agnes* (1LAg1, 2LAg1, 4LAg1), *Lady worthy of great respect* (1LAg12), *most venerable Lady* (3LAg1), *your Excellency* (1LAg31), *your holiness* (1LAg31), *daughter/blood-sister of the most excellent/illustrious King of Bohemia* (1LAg1, 3LAg1);
(b) **esteem**: *esteemed/holy/poor virgin* (1LAg1, 1LAg8, 2LAg18), *spouse/mother/sister of Jesus Christ/King of Kings/most high King of the Heavens/Lamb of the eternal King/the high King* (1LAg12, 1LAg24, 2LAg1, 3LAg1, 4LAg1, 4LAg4, 4LAg7, 4LAg15, 4LAg17), *handmaid of the Lord of Lords* (2LAg1), *very distinguished/noble/illustrious queen* (2LAg1, 2LAg20, 4LAg1, 4LAg15), *queen of the heavenly King* (4LAg27), *diligent imitator of the Father/poverty* (2LAg4, 2LAg7), *joy of the Angels* (3LAg11), *crown of the sisters* (3LAg11);
(c) and (c) **care**: *most beloved/dearest sister* (1LAg12, 2LAg24), *sister in Christ* (3LAg1), *dearest one* (3LAg10, 3LAg40), *most beloved in Christ* (3LAg11), *special/dearest/blessed daughter* (4LAg1, 4LAg17, 4LAg36, 4LAg39), *mother and daughter* (4LAg4).

Clare's selfless attitude and esteem for her follower, evident in her letters, seem to fit Winston's (2002, p. 5) and Patterson's (2003, p. 3) construct of agapáo love.

The virtuous construct of humility in servant leadership is described by Patterson (2003, pp. 3–4) as the ability to focus on others, not be arrogant, and keep one's accomplishments in perspective. Clare uses precise terms when she describes herself in the letters to Agnes, contrasting her lofty language in referring to her follower (see Table 7.3). She provides **no aristocratic title** for herself—even though, like Agnes, she came from an aristocratic family. She simply calls herself **Clare** (1LAg2, 2LAg1, 3LAg2, 4LAg2). She presents herself as:

Table 7.3 Repetitive-progressive pattern illustrating Clare's self-reference.

First Letter		*Second Letter*		*Third Letter*		*Fourth Letter*	
1LAg2	Clare an unworthy servant useless handmaid her subject servant in all things	2LAg1	Clare handmaid	3LAg2	Clare most humble unworthy handmaid servant	4LAg1	mother
		2LAg2	useless and unworthy handmaid			4LAg2	Clare unworthy servant useless handmaid handmaids
1LAg33	Your servant, though unworthy					4LAg33	poor little mother

the **servant of Agnes** (1LAg2, 1LAg33, 3LAg2, 4LAg2),
a subject (1LAg2),
handmaid (1LAg2, 2LAg1, 2LAg2, 3LAg2, 4LAg2),
unworthy/useless (1LAg2, 1LAg33, 2LAg2), 3LAg2, 4LAg2),
and **most humble** (3LAg2).

If Clare must take a leadership position regarding Agnes, she uses the descriptors of **mother and poor little mother** (4LAg1, 4LAg33). Clare's use of humble references to herself in the letters to Agnes keeps the focus on her follower. It is all about the follower in her letters. This deprecating self-referencing seems to suggest that humility is one of Clare's cardinal leadership values.

Patterson (2003, p. 4) describes altruism as serving others for the sake of serving, as radical equality and seeking the fulfillment of others. Clare's repetitive references to herself (see Table 7.3) as **unworthy/useless servant/handmaid** (1LAg2, 1LAg33, 2LAg2, 3LAg2, 4LAg2) further serve to communicate a radical, if not extreme, equality between leader and follower. The nature of this equality is expressed in the leader being a **subject** (1LAg2) and **servant in all things** (1LAg2) to the follower. Clare seeks Agnes' fulfillment and joy. She wants Agnes to embrace poverty (see Table 7.4) because it is a **"laudable exchange"** (1LAg30). This pursuit of poverty will lead to Agnes receiving and possessing **"blessed and eternal life"** (1LAg30). The humble attitude of Clare, a relationship of equality, and the desire to see Agnes blessed and fulfilled are reminiscent of the virtuous construct of altruism as described by Patterson (2003, p. 4).

The construct of vision in servant leadership is described by Patterson (2003, pp. 4–5) as a determined focus on the follower while providing the follower with a vision that will give the follower "purpose, direction, and dignity." Clare's vision can be described in one word: poverty (see Table 7.5). For Clare, the mystery of poverty is essentially part of the mystery of salvation and the Gospel (Ledoux, 1997, p. 55). Christ emptied Himself (*Philippians* 2:5–11) and became poor "so that people who were in utter poverty and want and in absolute need of heavenly nourishment might become rich in Him by possessing the kingdom of heaven" (1LAg20). Ledoux (1997, p. 54) links Clare's understanding of the poverty of Christ to her proclamation of the Lordship of Christ: "The Lordship of Jesus emerges from His poverty.

Table 7.4 Progressive pattern illustrating Clare's reference to the "laudable exchange" of poverty in the first letter to Agnes.

First Letter	
1LAg30	What a great laudable exchange: to *leave* the things of time for those of eternity, to *choose* the things of heaven for the goods of earth, to *receive* the hundred-fold in place of one, and to *possess* a blessed and eternal life.

Table 7.5 Repetitive-progressive pattern illustrating Clare's references to poverty.

First Letter		*Second Letter*		*Third Letter*		*Fourth Letter*	
1LAg6	holy poverty	2LAg2	the Poor Ladies utmost poverty	3LAg2	the Poor Ladies	4LAg18	blessed poverty
1LAg13	most holy poverty the Poor Crucified	2LAg7	holiest poverty	3LAg4	the poor and humble Jesus Christ	4LAg19	the poverty of Him
1LAg15	blessed poverty	2LAg18	poor virgin the Poor Christ	3LAg7	the arms of poverty	4LAg20	O astonishing poverty!
1LAg16	holy poverty			3LAg25	poverty in your chaste and virginal body,	4LAg22	His blessed poverty
1LAg17	God-centered poverty					4LAg33	poor little mother
1LAg19	the poor in this world						
1LAg20	utter poverty						
1LAg22	poverty						
1LAg25	the poor						

Our salvation, which is linked to this lordship, comes from Christ's abasement: Christ the Lord comes from the poor Christ." Clare describes Gospel poverty as:

(a) **holy** (1LAg6, 1LAg13, 1LAg16, 2LAg7),
(b) **blessed** (1LAg15, 4LAg22),
(c) **utter/utmost** (1LAg20, 2LAg2),
(d) **astonishing** (4LAg20),
(e) and (e) **God-centered** (1LAg17).

Agnes is encouraged by Clare to embrace Jesus, who is described as:

(a) **the Poor Crucified** (1Lag13),
(b) **the poor Christ** (1LAg18),
(c) and (c) **poor and humble** (3LAg4).

As Agnes embraces poverty, she will be a "**poor virgin**" (2LAg18), one of the "**poor ladies**" (2LAg2, 3LAg2), and so follow the example of her leader, who is a "**poor little mother**" (4LAg33).

Clare communicates a vision/charism of voluntary poverty that will enable Agnes to imitate the poor Christ and, in doing so, attain Christian perfection: "**chaste**" and "**pure**" (1LAg8). These theological elements in Clare's letters become Agnes' vocational vision. There is value congruence between Patterson's (2003, pp. 4–5) construct of vision and Clare's focus on Gospel poverty.

Patterson (2003, p. 5) describes the value of trust in servant leadership as closely aligned to the values of integrity and honesty that lead to credibility. The relationship between Clare and Agnes is one of radical equality. Clare not only plays the role of leader but also entrusts her vision and mission to Agnes, whom she describes as "the other half of her soul" (4LAg1). A repetitive-progressive pattern emerges when Clare's petitions for prayer from Agnes are examined in her letters (see Table 7.6). Clare petitions Agnes six times for prayers (1LAg33, 1LAg35, 2LAg26, 3LAg42, 4LAg37, 4LAg39). These petitions serve, amongst other things, to engender trust in Agnes. A reciprocal relationship of trust and equality is communicated through the use of this rhetorical device. A cursory reading of Clare's letters to Agnes shows that the relationship between her and her follower is not one of dominance but one of trust and integrity.

The construct of empowerment in servant leadership is described by Patterson (2003, p. 6) as the willingness to entrust followers with power, leading them to personal transformation as they act on their values. Agnes started her religious vocation with the option of virginity when she rejected the political marital alliances made for her by her father and communicated her desire for a celibate, consecrated life (Armstrong and Brady, 1982, p. 189). Mueller (2003, pp. 12–15) points towards the apparent connections between the life of Agnes and the legend of St. Agnes of Rome, who was martyred for her virginity in the Church's early years. Clare strengthens Agnes' resolve and option of celibacy by providing her with a theological foundation for her choice (see Table 7.7). Clare describes Agnes' virginity as:

(a) **holy** (1LAg1, 4LAg8),
(b) **prudent** (4LAg38),
(c) **to be esteemed** (1LAg1),
and (d) **inviolable** (1LAg13).

Table 7.6 Repetitive-progressive pattern illustrating Clare's petition for prayer.

First Letter		*Second Letter*		*Third Letter*		*Fourth Letter*	
1LAg33	I also beg You in the Lord, as much as I can, to include in Your holy prayers me	2LAg26	as often as possible, please remind your sisters to pray for us	3LAg42	and be sure to remember both me and my sisters in your holy prayers	4LAg37	please ask them to pray for me and my daughters in Christ
1LAg35	pray for me					4LAg39	pray for us

Table 7.7 Repetitive-progressive pattern illustrating Clare's references to virginity.

First Letter		*Second Letter*		*Third Letter*		*Fourth Letter*	
1LAg1	esteemed and most holy virgin	2LAg18	poor virgin	3LAg17	the Virgin a virgin	4LAg3	most holy virgins
1LAg7	your virginity	2LAg24	glorious Virgin of virgins	3LAg25	your chaste and virginal body	4LAg8	most holy virgin
1LAg8	virgin					4LAg38	the most prudent virgin
1LAg13	inviolable virginity						
1LAg19	the Virgin						
1LAg24	the glorious Virgin						

Agnes is encouraged to imitate the virginity of Mary, who is described as:

(a) **the Virgin** (3LAg17),
(b) **the glorious Virgin** (1LAg24),
(c) and (c) **the glorious Virgin of virgins** (2LAg24).

Clare empowers Agnes to act on her inherent belief that obedience to God means a celibate vocation for her.

Patterson (2003, p. 6) describes the "core" construct of service in servant leadership as the voluntary choice of the interests of others over self-interest. Clare refers to herself consistently as a **servant/handmaid/subject** (1LAg2, 1LAg 33, 2LAg1, 2LAg2, 3LAg 2, 4LAg2) that is **unworthy/useless** (1LAg2, 1LAg33, 2LAg2, 3LAg2, 4LAg2). Agnes is encouraged by Clare to accept this vocation of service that she describes as **holy** (1LAg13, 1LAg31). The repetitive-progressive pattern (see Table 7.8) illustrating Clare's references to service in the letters to Agnes serves to identify service as primary to Clare's understanding of leadership.

Kenotic Mysticism and Servant Leadership in the Letters of Clare of Assisi to Agnes of Prague

Clare links her vocation to service with a mystical attraction to Christ, who emptied Himself for others (see Table 7.9). Clare's desire to serve and hope to facilitate a similar spiritual formation in Agnes is fueled by "an ardent desire for the Poor Crucified" (1LAg13).

Both Francis and Clare were taken by the kenosis of Christ. Not only were they enthralled by this vision of the "poor Christ" (2LAg18), but they sought to imitate Him. Karecki and Wroblewski (2000a, pp. 12–13) write of Francis of Assisi:

Table 7.8 Repetitive-progressive pattern illustrating Clare's references to service.

First Letter		*Second Letter*		*Third Letter*		*Fourth Letter*	
1LAg2	an unworthy servant useless handmaid her subject servant in all things	2LAg1 2LAg2	handmaid useless and unworthy handmaid	3LAg2	unworthy handmaid servant	4LAg2	unworthy servant useless handmaid handmaids
1LAg4	all who serve seek to serve						
1LAg13	holy service						
1LAg26	serve served						
1LAg31	holy service						
1LAg32	serve						
1LAg33	Your servant, though unworthy						

Table 7.9 Repetitive-progressive pattern illustrating Clare's reference to service through kenotic mysticism in the first letter to Agnes.

First Letter	
1LAg13	Be strengthened in the holy service which You have undertaken out of an ardent desire for the Poor Crucified
1LAg31	be strengthened in His holy service

> In the kenosis of Christ, Francis saw God's infinite love for men and women in the condescension of the word in becoming human and laying down His life in Calvary. This coming down, this humbling, this stooping to become small, this humility and poverty, this minority was appropriated by Francis when he gradually stripped himself of all signs of power and status to identify with the poorest, the lepers.

Clare had the same vision. For Clare, "following in His footsteps" (2LAg7) were steps of love. Karecki (2000a, p. 2) comments:

> The Christ who captivated Clare's heart was the poor, suffering Christ and in response she consented to become His spouse. This is not an abstract image or concept, but a person, the person of Christ. Clare's poetic words to Agnes reveal a spousal intimacy that filled her with love.

This active contemplation of Jesus Christ is the way for Clare's transformation. Note the three-fold progression of terms (**loved, touched, accepted**) that are used in her first letter to Agnes (1LAg8) to describe the nature of the transformation: chaste, pure, virgin (Table 7.10). Another three-fold progression (**place your mind, place your soul, place your heart**) is evident in Clare's third letter to Agnes as she describes the transformative nature of Christo-centric contemplation (see Table 7.11).

The kenotic mysticism of Clare is rooted in a mimetic reenactment of the self-emptying—kenotic—Christ, as seen in the Christological hymn of *Philippians* 2:5–11 (Kourie, 1993, p. 127). This self-emptying becomes the hermeneutical key for Clare in interpreting the birth, life, death, and resurrection of Jesus Christ and applying its meaning to her community and her time (Kourie, 1993, p. 127). Christ is a mirror for Clare—or, as the Franciscan

Table 7.10 Progressive pattern illustrating Clare's reference to active contemplation in the first letter to Agnes.

First Letter	
1Lag8	When You have *loved* [*Him*], You shall be chaste; when You have *touched* [*Him*], You shall become pure; when You have *accepted* [*Him*], You shall be a virgin.

Table 7.11 Progressive pattern illustrating Clare's reference to active contemplation in the third letter to Agnes.

Third Letter	
3LAg12	*Place your mind* in the mirror of eternity; *Place your soul* in the splendor of glory;
3LAg13	*Place your heart* in the figure of the divine substance; And, through *contemplation*, **transform your entire being** **Into the image of the Divine One himself**,
3Lag14	So that you, yourself, may also experience what his friends experience When they taste the hidden sweetness That God alone has kept from the beginning For those who love him.

Brother Leo would call it, the *speculum perfectionis*; and she encourages Agnes to gaze into this mirror daily (4LAg 14–27; see Table 7.12). Note again the threefold progression in Clare's instruction of active contemplation in the fourth letter to Agnes: **look closely, consider, ponder**. As Agnes considers the voluntary poverty evident in Christ's birth, life, and death, she is encouraged to burn intensely with the "fire of charity" (4LAg 27). It is essential to note the choice of the metaphor of the mirror and the transformative dynamics it communicates. This kenotic metaphor is highly reminiscent of similar imagery in Paul's Second Letter to the Corinthians (3:18). For Clare, contemplation brings transformation that enables leaders to imitate and reflect God's virtues. Purfield (1989, p. 74) comments:

Table 7.12 Progressive pattern illustrating Clare's reference to active contemplation in the fourth letter to Agnes.

Fourth Letter	
4LAg14	Because the vision of him is the splendor of everlasting glory, The radiance of everlasting light, and **a mirror** without tarnish.
4LAg15	Look into **this mirror** every day, O queen, spouse of Jesus Christ, And continually examine your face in it,
4LAg18	Moreover, in **this mirror** shine blessed poverty, holy humility, and charity beyond words, as you will be able, with God's grace, to contemplate throughout the entire mirror.
4LAg19	Look closely, I say, to the *beginning of the life of this admired one*, indeed at the poverty of him who was wrapped in swaddling clothes and placed in a manger.
4LAg22	Consider also the midst of his life, his humility, or at least his blessed poverty, the countless hardships, and the punishments that he endured for the redemption of the human race.
4LAg23	Indeed, ponder the final days of this mirrored one, contemplate the ineffable love with which he was willing to suffer on the tree of the cross and to die there a kind of death that is more shameful than any other.
4LAg27	Therefore, seeing this, O queen of the heavenly King, you must burn ever more strongly with the fervor of charity!

> Clare reminds us that contemplation is not a mere reflection but, rather, it is a participation and a transformation of the beholder. She emphasizes that as they are being transformed, Christians, in turn, have to become mirrors and to reflect God.

Jesus is the paradigm and exemplar for Clare (Karecki and Wroblewski, 2000b, p. 12). The kenosis of Christ is the primary act of God's love for the world. Agnes is encouraged to make the kenosis of Christ her focus as she desires to serve (see Table 7.13)—again following Clare's three-fold progression of active contemplation in the second letter to Agnes: **gaze, examine, and contemplate**. This understanding of Divine Love leads to self-sacrificial service. Karecki and Wroblewski (2000a, pp. 12–13) comment: "Rarely is it pointed out that the genius of Francis and Clare's charism is that they made kenosis the special hallmark of Divine Love…What kenosis shows and clearly demonstrates is that Divine Love is non-possessive, disinterested, self-giving."

Kenotic mysticism allows the leader to transcend narrow selfhood (Kourie, 1993, p. 124) and genuinely enter the follower's world. Raguin (1973, p. 111) describes this state as receptive, noting:

> kenosis, then, places us in a state of receptivity. We develop an instinctive attitude of listening, trying to understand, letting ourselves be permeated with the atmosphere of our surroundings, passing beyond what is merely heard and seen to reach the personality of the people with whom we love, or those we may meet.

Kenotic mysticism in Clare's letters to Agnes is a direct communion with the kenotic Christ. Ledoux (1997, p. 40) notes: "in Clare's view, Christian mystical

Table 7.13 Progressive pattern illustrating Clare's reference to active contemplation in the second letter to Agnes.

Second Letter				
2Lag20	Gaze upon,			
		examine,		
			contemplate, most noble queen,	
				desiring to follow your spouse, who is more beautiful than the sons of humankind, and who for your salvation became the vilest of men, despised, struck, and flogged repeatedly over his entire body, dying while suffering the excruciating torments of the cross.
2Lag 21	If you *suffer with Him*, with Him you will **reign**,			
		grieving with Him, with Him you will **rejoice**,		
			dying with Him on the cross of tribulation, with him you will possess mansions in heaven among the splendors of the saints,	

experience achieves an encounter, a knowledge of and an existential communion with Christ." This communion with Christ leads to the personal transformation of the leader and follower and enables them to practice kenosis—self-emptying—as Christ did. This "resolute divesting" of possessions and power (Cronin, 1992, p. 1) allows the leader and follower to enter a new union marked by equality and service. Raguin (1973, p. 112) writes: "kenosis, then, is the gateway to mutual understanding, and beyond this, to an intimate sharing that is the consummation of a relationship in union...By dispossession of self, we are able to absorb the amazing riches of others." It is the resolute mimesis of the kenotic Christ that is the ground, expression, and consummation of Clare's spiritual direction that she offers Agnes. As Clare has found her deepest identity in Christ-centered poverty, she models and advocates this way of kenotic reenactment of the "Poor Crucified" (1 Lag13) as the way to the "blessed and eternal life" (1 LAg30).

Kenotic mysticism and servant leadership are closely linked in Clare's writings and her approach to spiritual direction in an interdependent dynamic system of personal and communal transformation through radical self-emptying fueled by a commitment to Jesus Christ. Successive repetitive-progressive pattern analyses of the letters of Clare of Assisi to Agnes of Prague suggest the following. Firstly, Greenleaf's (1998) description and Patterson's (2003) theoretical model of servant leadership fit the leadership approach and values of Clare of Assisi. Secondly, Clare links her kenotic mysticism with her practice of servant leadership and spiritual direction. Her "ardent desire" for the "Poor Crucified" brings her to service and forms the ground of her direction to her followers. However, more than a description of pious devotion, it is in this desire to emulate the poverty of Jesus that Clare finds her identity. Like the Apostle Paul, Clare's most frequent interlocuter, her private and social identity is formed by her desire to "know Him" (*Philippians* 3:10) in His poverty and condescension. Barentsen (2018, p. 4), in utilizing the interpretative lens of social identity theory, describes the Apostle Paul's leadership claim: "Paul turns accusations that his suffering disqualifies him from leadership on their head, arguing that faithful leadership must embody the sufferings of Christ in self-sacrificial forms of leadership rather than relying on status, patronage, and privilege." In a world driven mad by constant drives to climb the heights of power, privilege, and prestige, Clare models a radical vision and spiritual direction for Agnes, guided by her "ardent desire for the Poor Crucified": when she gazes, considers, contemplates, and imitates Christ, she will find her most profound and most authentic self. This mimetic reenactment of Christ brings healing and wholeness to Agnes and, ultimately, her world. Clare's Christ-centered direction to Agnes offers an alternative model for contemporary spiritual directors. Contemplation and appropriation of the kenosis of Christ enable the director and the one directed to transcend a narrow vision of self and facilitate a radical commitment to others in transformative service.

Notes

1 This chapter is based on initial arguments made in a presentation at the International Medieval Congress in 2008, entitled "*Iconic leadership: Kenotic mysticism and servant leadership in the Letters of Clare of Assisi to Agnes of Prague*," and in Bekker, C. J. (2013). Kenotic Mysticism and Servant Leadership in the Letters of Clare of Assisi to Agnes of Prague. *International Journal on Spirituality and Organization Leadership*. Volume 1, Issue 2, pp. 17–49. In both instances, these materials are used with permission from the author and publication.

2 For this chapter, all references to the Letters of Clare to Agnes are from Armstrong and Brady (1982) and will follow the convention of 1LAg13 meaning "First Letter to Agnes" line 13.

References

Alter, R. (1981). *The Art of Biblical Narrative*. Basic Books.

Armstrong, R. J. and Brady, I. C. (Eds. and Trans.). (1982). *Francis and Clare: The Complete Works*. Paulist Press.

Barentsen, J. (2018). The Social Construction of Paul's Apostolic Leadership in Corinth. *Hervormde Teologiese Studies* 74(4), 1–13.

Bekker, C. J. (2013). Kenotic Mysticism and Servant Leadership in the Letters of Clare of Assisi to Agnes of Prague. *International Journal on Spirituality and Organization Leadership*, 1(2), 17–49.

Bekker, C. J., and Burchard, M. A. (2015). Sequi Vestigia Christi: Aesthetic Hermeneutics and the Process of Leadership Conversions. *International Journal on Spirituality and Organization Leadership*, 3(2), 3–25.

Bekker, C. J. (2021). Sharing in the Incarnation: Towards a Model of Mimetic Christological Leadership. *International Journal on Spirituality and Organizational Leadership*, 1–21.

Bodo, M. and Sing, S. S. (1996). *On Retreat with Francis and Clare of Assisi – Following our Pilgrim Hearts*. St. Paul's Press.

Butler, D. C. (2003). *Western Mysticism*. Dover Publications.

Cai, W. (2022). St. Clare of Assisi and St. Agnes of Prague: Their Lives Intertwined by the Four Letters. Proceedings of the 2022 3rd International Conference of Mental Health, Education and Human Development . *Advances in Social Science, Education and Humanities Research*, 670, 1–3.

Carney, M. (1993). *The First Franciscan Women: Clare of Assisi and Her Form of Life*. Franciscan Press.

Chatman, S. (1978). *Story and Discourse: Narrative Structure in Fiction and Film*. Cornell University Press.

Cronin, K. M. (1992). *Kenosis*. Element.

Cunningham, L. S. (2004). *Francis of Assisi*. William B. Eerdmans Publishing Company.

De Beaugrande, R. A. and Dressler, W. U. (1981). *Introduction to Text Linguistics*. Longman.

De Robeck, N. (1954). *Saint Elizabeth of Hungary*. The Bruce Publishing Company.

Duw, T. M. (1992). *Saint Clare: A Light on the Way*. Catholic Truth Society.

Freeman, G. P. (2019). With Swift Pace and Light Step: On the Leadership of Clare of Assisi. *Franciscan Studies*, 77, 1–29.

Gerundt, M. and Warode, M. (2018). How Saint Clare of Assisi Guided Her Sisters: Impulses for Today's Leadership Context. *Religions* 9(347), 1–14.
Gowler, D. B. (1994). The development of socio-rhetorical criticism. In V. K. Robbins with D. B. Gowler (Eds.), *New boundaries in old territory: Form and social rhetoric in Mark* (pp. 1–35). Peter Lang.
Greenleaf, R. K. (1998). Servant-Leadership. In L. C. Spears (Ed.), *Insights on Leadership* (pp. 15–20). John Wiley and Sons.
Gregg, K. M. (2018). Clare of Assisi (1191–1253): Breaking through Societal Barriers for Women, in Denison. In B. J. Denison (Ed.). *Women, Religion, and Leadership: Female Saints as Unexpected Leaders* (pp. 33–55). Routledge.
Karecki, M. (2000a). *Clare and Christ*. The Little Portion. The Franciscan Institute of Southern Africa.
Karecki, M. (2000b). *The Generosity of God*. The Little Portion. The Franciscan Institute of Southern Africa.
Karecki, M. and Wroblewski, S. (2000a). *Franciscan Spirituality: Franciscan Study Guide Series*: Volume I. The Franciscan Institute of Southern Africa.
Karecki, M. and Wroblewski, S. (2000b). 2000B. *Franciscan Spirituality: Franciscan Study Guide Series*: Volume II. The Franciscan Institute of Southern Africa.
Karecki, M. and Wroblewski, S. (2000c). *Franciscan Spirituality: Franciscan Study Guide Series*: Volume III. The Franciscan Institute of Southern Africa.
Karecki, M. and Wroblewski, S. (2000d). *Franciscan Spirituality: Franciscan Study Guide Series*: Volume V. The Franciscan Institute of Southern Africa.
Karecki, M. and Wroblewski, S. (2001). *Franciscan Mission – The World is our Cloister: Franciscan Study Guide Series*: Volume I. The Franciscan Institute of Southern Africa.
Karecki, M. and Wroblewski, S. (2003a). *The Second Order: Franciscan Study Guide Series*: Volume I. The Franciscan Institute of Southern Africa.
Karecki, M. and Wroblewski, S. (2003b) *The Second Order: Franciscan Study Guide Series*: Volume V. The Franciscan Institute of Southern Africa.
Kourie, C. (1993). The Kenotic Mysticism of Clare of Assisi in the Light of Inter-religious Dialogue. *S.A. Journal of Medieval and Renaissance Studies* 3(1), 124–140.
Ledoux, C. (1997). *Clare of Assisi*. St Anthony Messenger Press.
Molesky-Poz, J. (2017). Saint Clare of Assisi: "May You Go Forward Securely." *Journal of World Christianity*, 7(1), 9–27.
Mooney, C. M. (2016). *Clare of Assisi and the Thirteenth Century Church: Religious Women, Rules, and Resistance*. University of Pennsylvania Press.
Mueller, J. (2003). *Clare of Assisi: The letters to Agnes*. Liturgical Press.
Neirynck, F. (1972). *Duality in Mark: Contributions to the Study of Markan Redaction*. Bibliotheca Ephemeridum Theologicarum Lovaniensium, XXXI. Leuven University Press.
Patterson, K. (2003). *Servant Leadership: A Theoretical Model*. Unpublished paper presented at the Servant Leadership Research Roundtable, Regent University.
Pecora, M. (2022). *Chiara: A Story of Saint Clare of Assisi*. Pauline Books and Media.
Pryds, D. (2012). Clare of Assisi. In M. A. Taylor and A. Choi (Eds), *Handbook of Women Biblical Interpreters: A Historical and Biographical Guide* (pp. 132–136). Baker Academic.
Purfield, B. E. (1989). *Reflections in the Mirror: Images of Christ in the Spiritual Life of Saint Clare of Assisi*. Unpublished Doctoral Dissertation at St. Bonaventure University, St. Bonaventure, New York.

Raguin, Y. (1973). *I am sending you (John 22:21): Spirituality of the Missioner.* East Asian Pastoral Institute.
Rimmon-Kenan, S. (1983). *Narrative Fiction: Contemporary Poetics.* Methuen.
Robbins, V. K. (1981). Summons and Outline in Mark: The Three-Step Progression. *Novum Testamentum* 23, 97–114.
Robbins, V. K. (1982). Mark 1:14–20: An Interpretation at the Intersection of Jewish and Graeco-Roman Traditions. *New Testament Studies*, 28, 220–236.
Robbins, V. K. (1984). *Jesus the Teacher: A Socio-Rhetorical Interpretation of Mark.* Fortress Press.
Robbins, V. K. (1987). The Women who touched Jesus' Garment: Socio-Rhetorical Analysis of the Synoptic Accounts. *New Testament Studies*, 33, 502–515.
Robbins, V. K. (1994a). *New Boundaries in Old Territory: Forms and Social Rhetoric in Mark.* Peter Lang.
Robbins, V. K. (1994b). Socio-Rhetorical Criticism: Mary, Elizabeth, and the Magnificat as a Test Case. In E. S. Malbon and E. V. McKnight (Eds.). *The New Literary Criticism and the New Testament* (pp. 164–209). Sheffield Academic Press.
Robbins, V. K. (1994c). The Ritual of Reading and Reading a Text as a Ritual: Observations on Mieke Bal's *Death and Dissymmetry.* In D. Jasper and M. Ledbetter (Eds.). *In Good Company: Essays in Honor of Robert Detweiler* (pp. 385–401). Scholars Press.
Robbins, V. K. (1994d). Interpreting Miracle Culture and Parable Culture in Mark 4–11. *Svensk Exegetisk Arsbok*, 59, 59–81.
Robbins, V. K. (1996a). *Exploring the Texture of Text. A Guide to Socio-Rhetorical Interpretation.* Trinity Press.
Robbins, V. K. (1996b). *The Tapestry of Early Christian Discourse. Rhetoric, Society and Ideology.* Routledge.
Scott, B. B. and Dean, M. E. (1993). A Sound Map of the Sermon on the Mount. *Society of Biblical Literature Society Papers*, 32, 726–739.
Tannehill, R. C. (1975). *The Sword of His Mouth.* Fortress Press.
Tannehill, R. C. (1989). *The Narrative Unity of Luke-Acts: A Literary Interpretation.* Fortress Press.
Trible, P. (1978). *God and the Rhetoric of Sexuality.* Fortress Press.
Trible, P. (1984). *Texts of Terror: Literary-Feminist Readings of Biblical Narratives.* Fortress Press.
Vorster, W. S. (1989). The Reader in the Text: Narrative Material. *Semeia*, 48, 21–39.
Winston, B. E. (2002). *Be a Leader for God's Sake.* Regent University.

Chapter 8

Engaging the Other in a Welcoming Space

Gordon Bermant

To be a spiritual companion—to engage in spiritual direction—requires frank encounters about truth, belief, faith, and fact. We cannot do this honestly unless both parties bring our histories, relationships, and the stories we tell to ourselves and others. Thus, at the risk of self-indulgence, with this essay I offer some stories about my heritage, history, and religious commitments in the interest of this chapter engaging in its own spiritual companionship to the reader. For me, this journey necessarily involves wading into Christian beliefs, the resurrection of Jesus in particular. In the face of that remarkable story, we will have to consider the methods of science and history as very specific ways many people attempt to verify or falsify asserted facts. Science and history are grounded in descriptions made according to institutional rules. However, religions, as we shall endeavor to show, go beyond such literal descriptions to reach for truths grounded in sensibilities and interpretations—not institutional rules. Religions, to the extent that they merit the name, propose truths that transcend ordinary categories to describe what is divine, absolute, and sacred. To speak and write religious truth, language must expand to include a wide range of figurative forms and styles. The word pointing to this category of language is *trope*. An easy example is that Jesus taught using parables. Parables are tropes. A parable may well use language that sounds historical or even scientific, but the goal for this type of trope is not to point to a historical or scientific fact, but to point beyond to the sort of truths with which religions ought to occupy themselves. The confusion regarding these matters gives rise to much pain and suffering.

Given the audacity of this undertaking, a fitting epigraph for the chapter is "forgive us our debts as we also have forgiven our debtors." We incur many debts to teachers, mentors, traditions, and friends. I certainly have accumulated many such debts on my journey. We also incur debts to our tropes, and we notice that the quoted prayer verse is itself a trope: a metaphor.[1] Thus, a seemingly simple enough transactional equation about forgiveness may open the possibility of deeper possibilities for meaning. For instance, who is the ultimate other to whom debts are owed? For many scholars and practitioners in Western history, Jesus Christ is the ultimate other. Jesus becomes this ultimate for such a broad range of

DOI: 10.4324/9781003742852-8

the world by virtue of the biblical and ecclesial accounts of his resurrection and ascension. And—whether as believers, dissenters, skeptics, or by mere exposure to those who are—hundreds of millions of people have been profoundly affected by the consequences of these accounts and how they are taken up.

Let us accept spiritual direction as a welcoming space where participants can shed straitjackets imposed by their linguistic histories. Participants come with their own meanings for what "spiritual" may mean for them; for many, it is an umbrella term intended to cover topics that are beyond the ordinary. Yet entering into territory beyond the ordinary demands some form of discernment if the process of spiritual direction is to have any shape or purpose. Thus, spiritual direction can also function as a forum addressing this question, central to this chapter: How are we to distinguish true claims from false claims in spiritual direction?

A cascade of follow-on questions might grow from this question. Here we will attend to two of them: How should we—directors and directees both—use the facts and methods of science to distinguish between true and false religious claims? How should we use the facts of history and the methods of historians to distinguish between true and false religious claims? That is, do these perspectives even belong in the space of spiritual direction? And if so, in what ways?

Readers are entitled to ask what qualifies me to write about this topic. The answer is nothing special. I am a retired old man who trained in psychology and in law and worked in jobs related to my training. My religious sentiments have been strong, yet my religious commitments took a long time to settle down.

A Brief Autobiography

I was born in Los Angeles in 1936, to parents who had driven there from Kansas 12 years earlier. My mother's maiden name was Wilson. Born in 1899, she was the youngest child of a family in Leavenworth, Kansas. She married my father in the early 1920s. Shortly thereafter, the couple drove across the great plains to settle in Los Angeles. A heavy smoker, she died of lung cancer in 1950, before my 14th birthday. My father was born in Junction City, Kansas in 1890. His father had emigrated to Kansas some years earlier from Metz, a city in France at its northeastern border with Germany. About the time the family left France for America in the early 1870s, France lost Metz to the new German Empire in the Franco-Prussian War. Metz became French again after Germany's defeat in World I. The Nazis turned the tables once more by annexing Metz into the Third Reich in 1940. The city became part of France yet again at the end of the war, and by 1950 Metz had become the principal city in the Moselle Department of the country, which it still is today.

I dwell on the location and history of Metz for one reason: I have come to the conviction that my paternal grandfather was a Jew. Why would I believe that? I was raised to believe that my family were Northern European Christians, with no biological or cultural Jewish connection. That was our story. I went regularly to Christian Science and Methodist Sunday schools and churches until 1957, when I moved to the East coast for graduate school.

Jews I met on the East coast told me they knew other Jews named Bermant. In the early 1960s, a Scottish Israeli who became a co-author and dear friend of mine, Julian Davidson (1931–2001), put me in touch with a friend of his, Chaim Bermant (1929–1998). Chaim Bermant was born in Latvia; his father was a rabbi. By the time I wrote to him in 1963, Chaim had already published widely on Jewish history and culture. He could not help me with names of Jews in Metz, but he assured me that our shared name was a Jewish one.

Several years ago, I sent a swab from my cheek to a DNA testing company. The report showed that my genotype is 25% Ashkenazi Jew. This is what I should expect if one of my four grandparents was fully Jewish but the other three were not. That result felt right to me. I am happy about it. Now I can characterize my mother's family as white bread and my father's family as white bread with Jewish jam. As to Metz, Jews have been there for more than a thousand years.

DNA genealogy has uncovered layers of many otherwise unknown stories. But it is fair to ask, So what? Who cares? Indeed. My Jewish genes are an enjoyable fact rather than a burden, unless I should have to flee antisemitic goons with murder on their minds—which I no longer believe cannot happen here. Regardless, history and science are already afoot as interpretive lenses and filters applied to my story about culture, influences, heritage, convictions, and all the many other facets of a life.

The public schools I attended in Los Angeles had large Jewish student populations. Fairfax High emptied out on Jewish holidays leaving only 40 of us *goyim* in classrooms, while the lucky Jews could celebrate Jewish holidays as they liked.[2] Over time, I learned that school was where I belonged and wanted to be. The result is that I have ended up doing bookish things in academic, government, and research institutions. I enjoy my books and my bookishness.

In graduate school during the late 1950s, becoming trained in the rigorous behaviorism of those days, I became a doctrinaire atheist, equating religion with superstition. A stroke of career luck took me to northern California for the decade of the 1960s. The atmosphere then and there began to melt my ice, as it did for many others as well. But it was not until 1986, after returning to the east coast to work, that I met a man who changed my life profoundly. His name was Kenryu T. Tsuji, a Canadian Japanese man born and raised in British Columbia. He became a minister in *Jodo Shinshu* Buddhism. Tsuji Sensei developed Shin Buddhist temples/churches[3] in Canada and then in the U.S. Eventually he settled with his wife and four daughters in Burke, Virginia, expanding the Shin Buddhist presence in this suburb of Washington, D.C. It was there, at Ekoji Buddhist Temple, that I met him, and with his guidance took refuge in Buddhism's Three Treasures. Reverend Tsuji died in 2004. For more about Tsuji Sensei, see my little book *Seeing What Is Already There* (Bermant, 2005).

This has been my religious trajectory: a beginning in Christianity, a personal discovery about Judaism, finally finding refuge in Buddhism. Much as one might share these broad strokes of one's journey early in spiritual direction, I share them with the reader. Thus, the rest of the chapter is organized in the same order: exploring several Christian responses to the challenge presented by the resurrection of Jesus; discovering a modern Jewish account of the resurrection that clarifies an important theological distinction; questioning religious claims under the standards of truth required by scientific and historical integrity; overall, emphasizing how tropes permeate religious texts and discourse; and finally, resting in a form of Mahayana Buddhism. Structurally, I would like to consider the extent to which these pivots and transformations may signify what can be an important journey in spiritual direction—moving from a desire to establish historical and scientific veracity, discovering the fundamental limits such pursuits reach, and finally coming to a very different sort of truth. Is this what spiritual direction is for everyone? I profoundly doubt it. It is, however, a major arc of my journey, facilitated through the spiritual direction I have received.

A Range of Responses to a Religious Challenge: The Resurrection of Jesus

Today there are approximately 8 billion people alive on earth, of whom 2.5 billion identify as Christian. About half of all Christians are Roman Catholics. Counting Protestant Christians is difficult because there are so many groups and sub-groups with diverse histories. The same holds for Orthodox Christian groups, which are usually named for their country of origin, for example Greek Orthodox, Russian Orthodox, Armenian Orthodox, and so on.

Like most religious identifications, not all Christians are reflective about their religious affiliation. But those who are thoughtful face a challenging question: how do they understand and express the crucifixion and resurrection of Jesus as the definitive events of Christianity?

The Bodily Resurrection of Jesus Three Days After His Crucifixion: Biblical Accounts

The biblical account of the Passion assures us that Jesus had died on the cross. His death is reported to Pontius Pilate by a Roman centurion. Pilate then allows Joseph of Arimathea to take Jesus down from the cross, wrap his body, carry the wrapped corpse to the tomb and place it there, then close the tomb and roll a large stone against the door (*Mark* 15:43–46). New Testament accounts of what happened next are astonishing: the body of the crucified Jesus had disappeared from this cave-like tomb by the time women who had been close to Jesus arrived to perform a ritual anointing of his corpse. Two alternatives to a miraculous resurrection were offered: a lie about robbery of the corpse by Jesus's followers at *Matthew* 28:11–15, and a fear expressed about professional grave robbers at

John 20:13; but these were falsified when Jesus appeared to the women and gave them specific instructions to pass along to his other followers.[4] With some variation, the women are identified as Mary Magdalene, Mary mother of James, and Salome. For the next 40 days,[5] Jesus is reported to have been seen by ever larger groups, until he ascended to Heaven to sit at the right hand of God.[6] The apostle Paul insisted on the fact of the bodily resurrection in his letter to new Christians in Corinth. The text of *1 Corinthians* 15:12–21 includes a stepwise argument exhorting them to accept it:

> Now if Christ is proclaimed as raised from the dead, how can some of you say there is no resurrection of the dead? If there is no resurrection of the dead, then Christ has not been raised; and if Christ has not been raised, then our proclamation has been in vain and your faith has been in vain. We are even found to be misrepresenting God, because we testified of God that he raised Christ—whom he did not raise if it is true that the dead are not raised. For if the dead are not raised, then Christ has not been raised. If Christ has not been raised, your faith is futile and you are still in your sins. Then those also who have died in Christ have perished. If for this life only we have hoped in Christ, we are of all people most to be pitied. *But in fact Christ has been raised from the dead, the first fruits of those who have died. For since death came through a human being, the resurrection of the dead has also come through a human being.*
>
> (Emphasis added, NRSV)

From the time of Paul's letter until today, his argument to a tragic conclusion, followed by a proclamation that tragedy is in fact averted, is among the most powerful statements of original Christianity. Paul urges the Corinthians not to give up on the truth of the resurrection as both physical and transcendent. Paul offers a truth and argument that he proclaims is essential to the life of the believer, and he does so with almost no literary ornamentation. An exception is in verse 20, "But in fact Christ has been raised from the dead, the first fruits of those who have died."[7] How shall we understand "first fruits" as a trope in this context?

The First Fruits: Literal and Metaphorical

Paul's exhortation is a masterpiece of unadorned argumentation. It is reasonable that he expected his readers to understand his use of "first fruits": no Corinthian, reading or hearing the impassioned text, would have wondered why Paul had inserted an agricultural term into a religious proclamation. Paul uses the term twice during this proclamation, when he writes "…for as all die in Adam, so will all be made alive in Christ. But each in his order: Christ the first fruits, then at his coming those who belong to Christ" (*1 Corinthians* 15:22–23). Then he fully develops the agricultural theme, challenging anyone who does not get the point:

> But someone will ask, "How are the dead raised? With what kind of body do they come?" Fool! What you sow does not come to life unless it dies. And as for what you sow, you do not sow the body that is to be, ...but a bare seed.... But God gives it a body as he has chosen, and to each kind of seed its own body. Not all flesh is alike, but there is one flesh for human beings, another for animals, another for birds, and another for fish.
>
> (35–39)

Paul makes two leaps: from agriculture to cosmology, then a profound leap into transcendence while retaining the agricultural language of process:

> There are both heavenly bodies and earthly bodies, but the glory of the heavenly is one thing and that of the earthly another.... So it is with the resurrection of the dead. What is sown is perishable, what is raised is imperishable. It is sown in dishonor, it is raised in glory.... Thus it is written, "The first man was from the earth, a man of dust; the second man is from heaven..."
>
> [F]lesh and blood cannot inherit the kingdom of God, nor does the perishable inherit the imperishable.... Listen! I will tell you a mystery! We will not all die, but we will all be changed...[T]he dead will be raised imperishable, and we will be changed. For this perishable body must put on imperishability, and this mortal body must put on immortality. When [this happens], then the saying that is written will be fulfilled: "Death has been swallowed up in victory. Where, O death, is your victory? Where, O death, is your sting?"
>
> (40–55)[8]

As we navigate these layers of imagery, perhaps we start to consider the implications of the tropes. Though modern English is comfortable with "perish" as a synonym of "die," we are uncomfortable, I think, with "perishable" as a synonym for the fate of an unpreserved corpse left to the elements.

First Fruits in Hebrew and Later Sources

A search of biblical text assures us that "First fruits"— בכורים [Heb. *Bikkurim*]—had been a familiar Jewish agricultural tradition/mitzvah for centuries.[9] Explicit uses of the term are found in more than 30 verses from *Exodus* to *Malachi*, and implicit references are present in numerous other Hebrew Testament locations. The term is shorthand for a *mitzvah* [a commandment (of kindness)] from God to the Jews that requires certain agricultural goods to be brought to the temple at a certain period of the year. *Leviticus* 23:9–14 quotes the language of the Lord to Moses with specific First Fruits requirements. Other verses are grouped to specify gifts to be made at several other religious festivals.

With one exception, the referents of First Fruits in these Hebrew Testament verses are agricultural and, thus, relatively literal. The exception is *Jeremiah* 2:3: "Israel was holy to the LORD, the first fruits of his harvest. All who ate of it were held guilty; disaster came upon them, says the LORD" (NRSV). This is the first Biblical use of the term as a metaphor.

References to First Fruits [Greek, ἀπαρχή, *aparché*] appear less frequently in the New Testament, but the phrase is used seven times, beginning in *Romans* and concluding in *Revelation*.[10] Advancing our observation that the New Testament authors turn literal expression in the Old Testament into tropes, we note that all of the seven uses are figurative. Paul, James, and John are no longer explaining the laws of the Torah; they are proclaiming new freedoms arising from faith in Jesus, using concepts familiar to their audiences.

To conclude: the trajectory of "first fruits" through the testaments, from mitzvah to metaphor, shows Christianity to be deeply embedded in the Jewish pastoralist and planter culture; yet, perhaps, participating in a shift in language and meaning.

The Body Old and New: Ecclesial Developments

Today, the bodily completeness of Jesus' resurrection remains affirmed and celebrated in Christian churches across the tradition: Roman Catholic, Eastern Orthodox, Lutheran, Presbyterian/Reform/Congregational, Latter-Day Saints, and newer American Bible-centered groups.[11] We can conclude that the body of Jesus affirmed in churches' teaching today is the same body of Jesus that the Bible reports was missing from its tomb on the third day after crucifixion and later appeared in the flesh to ever larger audiences. So, how do these various denominations make sense of this assertion?

Let Me Count the Reasons Why

Apologetic literature includes numbered lists of reasons for accepting the truth of the bodily resurrection. My survey of online sources turned up lists ranging from four to seven reasons. Even artificial intelligence has a confident answer. Microsoft's Bing answered my question "What reasons support the belief in the bodily resurrection of Jesus" with a list of four, including the claim that the growth of the Christian Church itself out of its Jewish context "in a brief window of time" was a compelling justification for faith in the bodily resurrection of Jesus.

The obedient reader of such explanations is still left, however, with some fundamental questions, not the least of which is, "what do I do with this as (a) truth?" In fact, one must do something with other truths as well if one is to make one's own sense of these truths. This is a not-unfamiliar impasse in spiritual direction as director and directee attempt to find what grounds the directee's life. One revered effort to thread this needle of truth comes from an august voice of 20th-century Protestant theology.

Rudolf Bultmann's Project to Demythologize Christianity, and Its Critics

Rudolf Bultmann (1884–1976), a Lutheran theologian who taught at the University of Marburg from 1921 until 1951, is well-known for his programmatic effort to separate the authentic message of the New Testament, the *kerygma* [κέρυγμα], from what he called the mythology embedded in the biblical texts and commentaries. The Greek *kerygma* translates to "proclamation"—for Bultmann: the historical truth conditions, rhetoric, and psychology associated with proclaiming, asserting, avowing. Bultmann's effort to dislodge *kerygma* from an ancient cosmology and reinstall it into a 20th-century worldview counts as an example of theology at work in a type of spiritual direction.

In 1941, Bultmann wrote an essay now regarded as one of the most influential theological documents of the mid-20th century. The original title is *Neues Testament und Mythos* (*New Testament and Mythology*). Readers unfamiliar with Bultmann may wonder, as I did, how a Christian theologian could function in the hell of atrocity-driven Germany during the Nazi era. In short, Bultmann resisted the Nazi use of Teutonic myths in his accounts of religious mythology in a way that avoided political reprisal.

New Testament and Mythology (1941) is still widely read, referenced, and debated.[12] Bultmann did not call for eliminating myth, but rather for interpreting it. He wrote that "The liberal theologians of the [nineteenth] century... threw away not only the mythology but also the *kerygma* itself" (Bultmann, 1961a, p. 16). This is a critical point of theological torsion. In this battle over types of truth, 20th-century reaction against 19th-century liberalism included reacceptance of mythology, but this was bound to discredit the truth of the New Testament in the minds of many people. Our worldview has become so influenced by the materialism of science and technology that we can no longer benefit from the truth of the *kerygma*. This is, after all, much of the struggle in spiritual direction as the directee yearns for a type of truth that may have been marginalized to the point of inaudibility. As a solution, Bultmann proposed adopting the existentialism of Kierkegaard and Heidegger. Bultmann called upon Christians to make an existential leap into an

> authentic life... based on unseen, intangible realities. Such a life means the abandonment of all self-contrived security. This is what the New Testament means by "life after the Spirit" or "life in faith." For this life we must have faith in *the grace of God.*
>
> (Bultmann, 1961a, p. 19)

How might we reflect on this exhortation within the welcoming space of spiritual direction? How might we understand authenticity for the directee who may only just be reaching some language to point to these "intangible realities"? We can ask for more guidance, with trail markers along our way.

Some of Bultmann's Christian critics objected that Bultmann's theology was too abstract and scholarly. Julius Schniewind (1961, p. 45) wrote that Bultmann's concerns were not unique to him and that "Every time we preach a sermon, we have to translate the language of the New Testament into the thought and language of the present day." He argued that Bultmann's concerns were legitimate, but that his solution was inadequate. Bultmann (1961b) took Schniewind's critique seriously enough to write a response addressed to it alone, in addition to his more general rejoinder to the other critics.

In his essay "The Right Interpretation of the Mythological," Ernst Lohmeyer (1961, p. 137) presented an interpretation of New Testament myth that rejects its elimination in favor of doubting "every sentence in the New Testament. Only under the pressure of doubt, doubt in everything and doubt in itself, can theology experience the triumphant power of its divine vocation." Philosophically and theologically rigorous as Lohmeyer's high-voltage proclamation may be, his stance would not be appreciated by parishioners seeking spiritual support in their Sunday sanctuaries. But in the quiet moments of spiritual direction, perhaps such pervasive doubt may find a place.

Further deepening the response to Bultmann, Helmut Thielicke (1961) provided a restatement of New Testament mythology. His goal was to refocus faith not on subjective experience of the myth, but rather on Jesus, the objective Christ. His concern was that the project of demythologizing can lead to weakening the power of the *kerygma*. Of prime importance is the event of the resurrection. Bultmann and Thielicke disagreed about the correct account of events on that day. Yet both of them wanted to prevent the weakening of faith. The two theologians thus shared a purpose but proposed opposing methods to achieve it.

Bultmann's fourth German critic, Friedrich Schumann summarized Bultmann's thesis beginning with the cosmological concept of antiquity that Bultmann wished to unseat:

> a three-storied universe consisting of heaven, earth, and the underworld; the intervention of natural and supernatural powers in human life; the dominion of evil powers and Satan over that life and also over the external realm of nature; the imminent end in time of this world-aeon.
> (Schumann, 1961, p. 175)

Schumann followed with Bultmann's proclamation of the good news of the New Testament:

> *now* is the time of the End here, for the Son of God appeared as a pre-existent cosmic being. His death brings deliverance from the bondage of sin and the power of Satan, his resurrection is the defeat of the power of

> death, his impending return will be the end of this aeon and the inauguration of the Kingdom of God, the judgment of this world and the perfection of the community of believers.
>
> (Schumann, 1961, p. 175)

Bultmann held that modern minds, trained in empiricism and scientific skepticism, could no longer accept the cosmology and miraculous interventionism of the ancient worldview. Schumann argued that Bultmann's solution was inadequate. Accepting the resurrection as an event in history is not to be rationalized through ignorance, for example that only those who were present at the time could have known for certain. Schumann insisted that the historical record must be interpreted affirmatively: "The gospel of Jesus Christ is not the communication of factual truths or neutral information, which may appeal to us or not. It is the communication of a decisive understanding of human experience" (Schumann, 1961, pp. 176–177). Nevertheless, the bind is that our modern worldview prevents acceptance of that understanding. And it is just here that Schumann finds Bultmann turning to Heideggerian existentialism as a necessary condition precedent to faith.

Schumann (1961) introduces the German term *Verfallen-Sein* [being in fallenness] to be the existentialist equivalent of universal human sinfulness that follows from the story of Adam, Eve, and snake. But the question remains whether this modern sense of fallenness can hold all the psychic implications forwarded by the entire biblical account of "original sin" including scripture from both Hebrew and New Testaments. In the Christian interpretation of that story, the only escape from the consequences of our sinfulness is acceptance of God's grace as uniquely proven through the crucifixion and resurrection of Jesus.[13]

Neither Schumann nor Bultmann went so far as to make a complete substitution of Heideggerian fallenness for biblical sinfulness. How Bultmann expressed this reservation against modernity is close to the core of his theology and his personal affirmation:

> Can the resurrection narratives and every other mention of the resurrection in the New Testament be understood simply as an attempt to convey the meaning of the cross? Does [the resurrection] not express this truth… that the Crucified was not holden of death but rose from the dead?
>
> Yes indeed: the cross and the resurrection form a single, indivisible cosmic event. "He was delivered up for our trespasses, and he was raised for our justification" (Romans 4:25). The cross is not an isolated event, as though it was the end of Jesus which needed the resurrection subsequently to reverse it. When he suffered death, Jesus was already the Son of God, and his death by itself was the victory over the power of death…. [T]he resurrection is not a mythological event

> adduced in order to prove the saving efficacy of the cross, but an article of faith just as much as the meaning of the cross itself. Indeed, *faith in the resurrection is really the same thing as faith in the saving efficacy of the cross.*
>
> (Bultmann, 1961a, pp. 38, 39, 41)

Bultmann also addressed the reality of the resurrection in the two volumes of *Theology of the New Testament* (Bultmann, 2007 [1948]). Here is a representative statement, from volume 2, in a section titled "The Salvation-Occurrence":

> Nothing preceding the faith which acknowledges the risen Christ can give insight into the reality of *Christ's resurrection.* The resurrection cannot—in spite of I Cor. 15: 3–8[14]—be demonstrated or made plausible as an objectively ascertainable fact on the basis of which one could believe. But insofar as it or the risen Christ is present in the proclaiming word, it can be believed—and only so can it be believed. Belief in the resurrection and the faith that Christ himself, yes God Himself, speaks in the proclaimed word (II Cor. 5:20)[15] are identical.
>
> (Bultmann, 2007 [1948], p. 305)

Finally and unequivocally, Bultmann proclaims that the crucifixion and resurrection, together, are the transcendent events that the biblical texts have promised: they mark the end of ordinary history by providing divine salvation through God's grace, available to humans "not by philosophical discussion, but only by faith and obedience" (Bultmann, 1961a, p. 44). They are completely real yet beyond proof. This proclamation is not based in myth, because in myth, transcendent events are "reduced" to immanent events. "Instead, we have the paradox of a transcendent God present and active in history: 'The Word became flesh'" (Bultmann, 1961a, p. 44).[16]

A Comment on Bultmann's Conclusion

I found the last quoted text to become frantic, as if Bultmann had searched for *more*, deep in the biblical text and personal commitments, to support an unambiguous affirmation of the historical truth of bodily resurrection—but could not find it. Of course, he was very well aware of Paul's warning of the dire consequences of denial, which Bultmann would not accept. He responded to the bind he was in by linking the resurrection as "a fact of the proclaiming word" with the historical reality of the crucifixion, thus creating "the paradox of a transcendent God present and active in history," a paradox that Christians must embrace with "faith and obedience."

Such are the challenges anyone who decides that they ought to enter into something like spiritual direction faces. Our thoroughly modern intellects face off with longings, convictions, cherished experiences. Though the language of these various arguments may, at times, seem distant from our experiences, Bultmann, his critics, and we are all still posed with these fundamental questions about truth and what sense to make of the tropes of our traditions.

The Jewish Perspective of Pinchas Lapide

Many original Christians were Jews. What was their religious context at the time of the crucifixion and resurrection?

Call it coincidence or call it synchronicity,[17] but I have been aided by the publication "A Jewish Theology of Resurrection," by Rabbi Mark Gottlieb (2023). Gottlieb described the work of Pinchas Lapide (1922–1997), a remarkable Austrian Israeli diplomat, theologian, and author. Among his many books, he published *Auferstehung: ein jüdisches Glaubenserlebnis* in 1978, which was translated and published in English paperback in 2002 as *The Resurrection of Jesus: A Jewish Perspective.*

Lapide shows that resurrection was not foreign to the Mosaic tradition, with at least three resurrections to be found in the Hebrew Testament.[18] In the New Testament, seven resurrections are reported.[19]

Lapide (2002) takes pains to emphasize the embeddedness of the apostles in their Judaic traditions. Paul called himself a Pharisee even after his transformative encounter with an image of Jesus while he, then Saul the zealous tax collector, was on the road to Damascus. In his self-defense address to King Agrippa, after the priests in Jerusalem had arrested and imprisoned him for his Christian proclamations, Paul said

> I have belonged to the strictest set of our religion and lived as a Pharisee. And now I stand here on trial on account of my hope in the promise made by God to our ancestors, a promise that our twelve tribes hope to attain, as they earnestly worship day and night. It is for this hope, your Excellency, that I am accused by Jews! *Why is it thought incredible by any of you that God raises the dead?*
>
> (Emphasis added, *Acts* 25: 5–8 NRSV)

The hope, of course, is for the arrival of the Messiah.

Lapide explains that the Pharisees accepted the reality of bodily resurrection, but the more conservative Sadducees did not. Acceptance of Jesus as Lord carried very serious additional complications: how were new Christians from among Jews to understand their new social and moral obligations? For example, were they still bound by the Mosaic ritual laws? And what about Gentiles who accepted the proclamations of apostolic Christians from among the Jews: must the Gentile men submit to circumcision and learn to follow Jewish rituals including dietary restrictions? This bundle of issues created conflict among the earliest Christians and continued to be unsettling for generations thereafter.

Paul's agonized question shows that the bodily resurrection of Jesus is consistent with the social imaginary of Pharisaic Judaism. He was exasperated that others around him failed to accept it. Lapide also allows himself an exasperated comment about theories of the resurrection developed in the 20th century by Roman Catholic and Protestant theologians. After giving several examples of their texts, Lapide says:

> Most of these and similar conceptions strike me as too abstract and scholarly to explain the fact that the solid hillbillies from Galilee who, for the very real reason of the crucifixion of their master, were saddened to death, were changed within a short period of time into a jubilant community of believers.... One thing we may assume with certainty: neither the Twelve nor the early church believed in the ingenious wisdom of theologians! ... I cannot rid myself of the impression that some modern Christian theologians are ashamed of the material facticity of the resurrection.
>
> (Lapide, 2002, pp. 129–130)

The first theologian on the list of those Lapide complained about was a famous one: Rudolf Bultmann.

Lapide traversed careful middle ground at the conclusion of the book. He can accept the physical resurrection of Jesus, but he does not accept that Jesus is the hoped-for Messiah:

> I therefore can accept neither the messiahship of Jesus for the people of Israel nor the Pauline interpretation of Jesus.... On the other hand, a dialogue between Jews and Christians can be carried out seriously only if the Jewish partner also starts out with the assumption that Christianity is a faith fellowship desired by God which concerns him "for God's sake," even if he does not see in it a way which he himself can or must go.... Without glossing over or bypassing the differences, a dialogue in which both partners take the faith substance of the other as seriously as their own could become a true dialogue—from open faith to open faith, from confidence to confidence... and from joy in the duality which knows its ultimate unity only in God.
>
> (Lapide, 2002, pp. 153–154)

It is just such a dialogue that we hope to be advancing here—the very dialogue that occurs in spiritual direction, even when the two parties affirm the same doctrines.

How Are We to Use the Facts of *Science*, and the Methods Scientists Use, to Distinguish True Claims from False Claims About the Resurrection of Jesus?

We have presented affirmations of the bodily resurrection of Jesus. How shall we evaluate these affirmations in the light of scientific methods and results?

I begin by describing a March 4th, 2013, *New Yorker* cartoon by David Sipress. God and an angel are sitting on a cloud while the angel reads a request to God from the day's mail: "Mrs. Marsha Mullhouse, of Kenosha, Wisconsin, asks 'Are you subject to the laws of physics, or are the laws of physics subject to You?'" This is a profound question. God sits chin on hand, pondering His response.

What if the cartoon is merely silly because God, as expressed in religions, is a fiction, a myth, a mistake? What if the laws governing the universe foreclose on the possibility of God and any other supernatural principle or process? In this view, the only true natural laws are the laws verified scientifically. God is a product of religion, which is a purely human product, a verbal invention, the ultimate trope. What if science and religion are incompatible, and science prevails?

I borrowed the term "incompatible" from the subtitle of a book written in the genre of so-called New Atheism. New Atheism is new primarily because its authors and their books gained a lot of public visibility in the first and second decades of this century. Particularly prominent in the first decade were: Richard Dawkins (*The God Delusion*, 2006); Daniel Dennett (1942–2024) (*Breaking the Spell*, 2006); Sam Haris (*Letter to a Christian Nation*, 2006); and Christopher Hitchens (1949–2011) (*God Is Not Great*, 2007). In 2019, these four published *The Four Horsemen: The Conversation That Sparked an Atheist Revolution*, based on a conversation they had recorded in 2007. Dawkins and Harris were trained to ride the horses of science; Dennett practiced analytic philosophy; and Hitchens was a gifted, persistent polemicist on a variety of topics.

In 2015, the evolutionary geneticist Jerry A. Coyne published *Faith vs. Fact: Why Science and Religion are Incompatible*. I prefer Coyne's book to the others because his humanity projects to the reader. Even an atheist can be a *mensch*. And if we are going to pursue spiritual direction—with or without God—we need humanity and *menschen*. There is in Coyne's book none of the sarcasm, smugness, and snark that saturated the stables of the horsemen. For all his humanity, however, Coyne is unsparing in his attack on religion. Before one turns a page of the main text for the first time, in the Preface, Coyne informs the reader that his thesis

> is that religion and science compete in many ways to describe reality… but use different tools to meet this goal. And I argue that the toolkit of science, based on reason and empirical study, is reliable, while that of religion—including faith, dogma, and revelation—is unreliable and leads to incorrect, untestable, or conflicting conclusions. Indeed, by relying on faith rather than evidence, religion renders itself *incapable* of finding truth.
>
> (Coyne, 2015, xi–xii)

Coyne is at his best while deconstructing three "test cases" of religious claims: the original sin of Adam and Eve infected humans forever after, requiring the redemptive death of Jesus; Mormon teaching claimed the discovery in 1827 of scripturally-inscribed golden plates on Joseph Smith's farm in New York State; and creationists connected the doctrine of *imago Dei* to so-called theistic evolution, a historical process directed by God. Each of these faith-based human histories makes claims that are unsupportable to a degree that leaves but two choices for those who will not reject them: either accept them as myths or declare that the sources are inerrant.

Coyne (2015) does not shy away from discussing resurrection. While he does not accept bodily resurrection as a valid description of what happened to the body of Jesus on the third day, his scientific open-mindedness requires him to remain open about the possibility of a miracle: "It would be a closed-minded scientist who would say that miracles are impossible in principle" (Coyne, 2015, p. 124). This admission comes after pages of argument against the efforts of theologians, historians, philosophers, and scientists—Stephen J. Gould in particular—to find a compromise that allows contradictory faith-based and science-based claims to co-exist, both as correct. Coyne rejects accommodation utterly—up to the limit of being closed-minded about it.

As we sit in this scientific paradigm, there is some philosophy that can be useful in illuminating the wall separating science from religion, which Coyne makes insurmountable: *there is more than one criterion of truth.*

Philosophers carefully delineate three kinds of truth: *correspondence, coherence*, and *pragmatic.* The truth that Coyne defends so skillfully against religion is truth as correspondence: a definite connection between something in the world and a statement naming or characterizing that something. We can understand science as rules for making definite connections and the results to date. Science shows how language will map or mirror the objects of the world. Some aspects of religion are subject to analysis and verification through correspondence, but not all of them. We can understand that the parables of Jesus, for example, are tropes rather than literal descriptions.

Religion can certainly aspire to the second category: truths of coherence. "A coherence theory of truth states that the truth of any (true) proposition consists in its coherence with some specified set of propositions" (Young, 2018 [1996] para. 1). The work is done in the language being employed; it need not reach out into objects in the world, as correspondence truth does. A religion is coherent when its terms fit sensibly together, so that implications based on some terms in the religion's vocabulary make sense when brought into connection with other terms of equally good standing in the religion's documents. This is the sense of truth that Christian scholar Richard Swinburne refers to in his book *The Coherence of Theism* (Swinburne, 2016 [1977]).

Third, very important in the current context, is the pragmatic theory of truth. "[P]ragmatic theories of truth tend to view truth as a function of the practices people engage in, and the commitments people make, when they solve problems, make assertions, or conduct scientific inquiry" (Capps, 2023 [2019], para. 1). Pragmatic truth theory included the contributions of William

James (1842–1910), America's greatest psychologist, who connected truth with utility: "what works." William James was also the author of *The Varieties of Religious Experience* (1902). Here again James catalogued "what works."

Reflecting on different forms of truth in respect to religious promises and commandments clarifies—but for many people does not resolve—the unique status of some religious claims. Many truth seekers still want to know: "Did it happen or not?" This is a question about history.

How Are We to Use the Facts of History, and the Methods Historians Use, to Distinguish True from False Claims in Spiritual Direction?

Coyne's (2015) anti-religion arguments are often historical rather than scientific. What is the difference? If we start with a historical claim, such as "Jesus arose from his grave on the third day after his crucifixion," we understand that there are two general ways to reject the claim, either by saying "No, He did not" or "No, He could not." The first rejection is simply historical: that event did not happen on that day in that place. The second rejection goes further: "No He did not, because He could not." But the reverse is not true: if Jesus did not arise from his grave on the third day after his crucifixion, it does not follow that he never did so, or could not have done so. Remember Coyne's statement that "It would be a closed-minded scientist who would say that miracles are impossible in principle" (Coyne, 2015, p. 124). Yet, something true in principle is not, for that reason alone, a historical fact. This creates a problem, doesn't it? This problem has taken the form of a particular ditch.

Lessing's Ditch

Now the conversation gets a bit more complicated. Bultmann and other theologians scrambled to find literal and figurative statements to support seekers' surrender to Christian faith. We tend to trust eyewitness accounts, and the scriptures report the fully resurrected Jesus being seen by increasing numbers of people. But these scriptural reports were written 30 years or more after the events they describe. The Gospels' authors were not investigative journalists. They were devout believers proclaiming the miracle of God, simultaneously human and divine, who had walked among their predecessors and then ascended to sit at the right hand of God the Father.

The inescapable problem of history was turned into a powerful metaphor in the eighteenth century by the German philosopher G. E. Lessing (1729–1781). Lessing's philosophical project was to make all knowledge rational. He found that Christianity, having long lost the immediate impact of the life of Christ on earth, could not rest on historical accounts, because all historical truths are accidental—could have been otherwise; but religious truths must be necessary—beyond doubt. He used a powerful trope to describe the gap between historical and necessary truth, calling it a *garstige breite Graben*, translated as "ugly broad ditch" or "nasty wide trench" that cannot be crossed. We have arrived—through theological reasoning, scientific methods, and historiography—at the ditch to which this trip has been headed. And we return to the existentialism of Kierkegaard and Heidegger for the trope that we need now: a *leap of faith* (that we encountered earlier used by Bultmann), to cross over the nasty trenches of historical uncertainty. Where does it land?

Is Japan East or West of Here? Finding Buddhism in a Northern Virginia Suburb

Earlier, I described my commitment to True Pure Land Buddhism—*Jodo Shinshu*. The English trope is to *take refuge* in Buddhism's Three Treasures: the Buddha, the Dharma, and the Sangha. Finding out what taking refuge means has been my religious exercise for almost 40 years. Along the way I have tried to explain my commitment to others (Bermant 2005, 2017a, 2017b). Here I begin with a strong claim: In an unusual but effective way, Jodo Shinshu bridges Lessing's ditch.

Here is how the trope makes sense.

The Pure Land tradition began in India several hundred years BCE and migrated over centuries through China, Korea, Japan, and into the United States at the end of the nineteenth century. There is a mountain of meticulous scholarship across Asian and Western languages about the True Pure Land tradition, but there is also an irony about that: the tradition has for centuries focused on the spiritual needs and competencies of everyday lay people rather than on renunciants or scholars.

The Larger Pure Land Sutra[20] (Inagaki and Stewart, 1994) tells the story of Dharmakara, a king who aspires to Buddhahood.[21] He is instructed by the Buddha Lokesvararaja to travel to the unique land of every other Buddha, who are more numerous than the grains of sand in the Ganges River, then report back about what he has learned. Dharmakara's fact-finding mission lasts five *kalpas*, which is in the order of five billion years. Upon his return, Dharmakara makes 48 vows for the benefit of all sentient beings, promising that if the vows are not fulfilled, he will renounce his desire for Buddhahood.

But the vows are fulfilled! And Dharmakara becomes *Amitabha/Amitayus—Amida* in Japanese Buddhism: the Buddha of Infinite Light and Life, Wisdom and Compassion, whose Buddha land, Sukhavati, in the far (!) West, is accessible at rebirth by those who have placed their trust in Amida and faithfully recite his name. Practice in this pure land for one lifetime allows nirvana for the practitioner, which is the termination of the otherwise endless repetition of deaths and births into yet another life of suffering.[22]

This foundational text presents a *fabulous* history, with miraculous events occurring over billions of years. There is no religious need to put this history on a calendar, because it is hyperbolically beyond any *possible* calendar. We are given a text that makes searching for historical truth no more than a fool's errand. We are invited to sit down, shut up, and pay attention to the world as it is. The sutra promises relief from existential dissatisfaction, but the guarantee has no date on it. If the promise is valid, I should be able to experience the benefits. My task is to recognize and appreciate a benefit when it comes my way, whether large or small. Rejecting the doctrine of multiple lifetimes is not a deal breaker.

I don't know what it would be like to believe the sutra as recounting an actual event in human history. And in my 37 years as a grateful Shin Buddhist who has met many other Shin Buddhists from "all corners of the globe"—a nonsensical trope if there ever was one—I have yet to meet an adult who confessed to a literal belief in it. It is literally beyond belief.

And yet… the figure of Amida Buddha, visualized, called for, and "heard calling," has comforted me and continues to comfort me, and I understand how this can be. The visualization is a trope, a personification of a metaphysical principle that is beyond visualization. What is this principle? It is *Sunyata*, "emptiness," *dharmakaya*, the nature of reality. Volumes have been written in reference to it, but it also leads serious people to say, "I open my mouth, I make a mistake." Better to remain quiet with an image and a posture. The image is wisdom and compassion personified: Amida Buddha. The posture is the gesture of *gassho:* palms together, fingertips held just below chin level. The gesture is a symbol, a non-verbal metaphor of non-duality. If moved to speak, announce the Buddha's name and contemplate these lines from the Shin Buddhist teacher Kenryu Tsuji:

> When I call Amida's name,
> It's Amida calling me.
> His voice and my voice are one.
> I gassho with Amida.

A transcendent Other and I, sounding together. I am at home in this space to contemplate spiritual direction (see Bermant, 2015). Thank you.

Notes

1 *Matthew* 6:12 (NSRV). The New Oxford Annotations of the NRSV tell us that "debts" is a metaphor for "sins" and "debtors" for "sinners." The annotators of the 1988 KJV concur with the sin-to-debt metaphor and say further that our sins "are our moral and spiritual debts to God's righteousness."
2 See Deborah Moore (1994).
3 There is no important difference between "church" and "temple" titles in North American Shin Buddhist locations for practice.
4 *Matthew* 28, *Mark* 16, *Luke* 24, *John* 20, *Romans* 5, 1 *Corinthians* 15, and 1 *Thessalonians* 4.
5 Readers with a fascination for numbers may remember that Moses and the Israelites wandered for 40 years in the Sinai Desert before Joshua led them into Caanan, the Promised Land. Is there something biblically *special* about the

number 40? I stood at the opening of this rabbit hole for a short while, aware that jumping into it would occupy me for more time than I had to give to it. I went in just far enough to know that I was right about that, as evidenced by the following summary from an Evangelical Fundamentalist Christian source: "The number 40 appears 146 times in the Bible, a number of God's significance. We think of Noah, of the years in the wilderness, of the days Moses was on the Mount, of Jonah and Nineveh, and, in Jesus' case, the number of days he was tempted of the devil…and the number of days between the Resurrection and the Ascension. Usually this number signifies testing, trials, probation, or a provision of prosperity. We must believe the last comes closest to the risen Lord's season before He ascended" (Marshall, n.d.).

6 Acts 1:9. The fundamental importance of the Ascencion of Jesus for the history of Christian organization is emphasized by Douglas Farrow, cited in the references.

7 Other translations often end the sentence with "sleeping" or "are asleep" rather than "dead." It is interesting to ask whether the reference to sleep rather than death is a literal claim or a trope (euphemism).

8 I am uneasy about my elisions of parts of Paul's magnificent rhetoric and urge readers to engage with the complete text of *1 Corinthians* 15.

9 See, for example, Bogomilsky (n.d.) and Jastrow and Friedländer (n.d.).

10

1. *Romans* 8:23. Though possessing the first fruits from the Spirit, new Christians "groan," waiting for the redemption of the body.
2. *Romans* 11:13–24. Speaking to Gentiles who have accepted Christianity, Paul uses agricultural terms to explain how the Gentiles relate to Jews who have become Christians. Although I confess to personal confusion with Paul's trope here, which seems to move from the first fruit of bread with the first fruit of a plant or tree.
3. *1 Corinthians* 15, 23: see above.
4. *1 Corinthians* 15, 23: see above.
5. *2 Thessalonians* 2:13. There is discussion among experts whether "first fruits" is a preferable translation to "has chosen you for salvation." In either case, there is no agricultural reference but rather an emphasis on God's—and Paul's—satisfaction with the new Thessalonian Christians.
6. *James* 1:18. Together with verse 17, James proclaims the true nature of God and explains to all Jews who have become Christians that they are a "kind of first fruits of [God's] creatures."
7. *Revelation* 14:4. John describes a vast group of virginal Christian men whose purity make them first fruits "unto" God and the Lamb.

11 For a quick range of resources: Catechism of the Catholic Church (1997), 638–658; Orthodox Wiki (2013); Harder (n.d.); Ensign-George (2021); White (n.d.); Mormon Wiki (n.d.). Nevertheless, there is not complete unanimity among the American Bible-centered churches. Jehovah's Witnesses, for example, teach that Jesus rose from death as a spiritual being. The First Church of Christ, Scientist accepts that the gospels proclaim the bodily resurrection of Jesus, while also proclaiming its own philosophical idealism such that all materialism is illusory.

12 Bartsch (1961, p. vii) notes in his introduction to a critical volume on the book, "No single work which has appeared in the field of New Testament scholarship during the war years has evoked such a lively discussion as Bultmann's original manifesto, '*New Testament and Mythology.*'"

13 See Keathley (2004).

14 Here is *1 Corinthians* 15:1–8 (NRSV): "For I handed on to you as of first importance what I in turn had received: that Christ died for our sins in accordance with the scriptures, and that he was buried, and that he appeared to Cephas, then to the twelve. Then he appeared to more than five hundred brothers and sisters at one time, most of who are still alive, though some have died. Then he appeared to James, then to all the apostles. Last of all, as to one untimely born, he appeared to me."

15 Here I quote *2 Corinthians* 5:20–21, which is the final verse of the chapter. "So we ambassadors for Christ, since God is making his appeal through us; we entreat you on behalf of Christ, be reconciled to God. For our sake he made him to be sin, who knew no sin, so that in him we might become the righteousness of God" (NRSV).

16 Bultmann here is quoting *John* 1:14: "And the Word became flesh and lived among us, and we have seen his glory, full of grace and truth." (NRSV).

17 I thank my friend Karen Blanc Friedman, who first told me about the "Pauli-Jung conjecture" on synchronicity, defined as "meaningful coincidence" or "acausal parallelism."

18 *1 Kings* 17:17–24; *2 Kings* 4:18–37; and 2 Kings 2:9–12.

19 Jesus performed three of these during his ministry (*Luke* 7:11–17, Jesus raises a dead boy; *Luke* 8:40–56, Jesus raises a dead girl; *John* 11:1–44, Jesus commands Lazarus to emerge from his tomb four days after his corpse had been sealed within). The resurrection of Jesus is reported, with varying details, at *Matthew* 28:1–10, *Mark* 16:1–7, *Luke* 24:1–49, and *John* 20:1–29. Peter and Paul each raise the dead once during their ministries (Acts 9:36–42, when Tabitha, aka Dorcas, is raised by Peter at her home in Joppa; and Acts 20:7–12, when Paul raises the young man Eutychus, who had fallen three stories to the ground).

20 Also known as the Longer Pure Land Sutra, which is the title given to it on Wikipedia.

21 The name Dharmakara is already a trope; it means storehouse of the sutras.

22 This sutra shares features with other Mahayana sutras: there are a multitude of Buddhas in the universe, each with a unique Buddha land. Sutras are formed as narratives by the historical Buddha, Siddartha Gautama. The sutra's author begins the text with the formulaic statement, "Thus have I heard," indicative of an oral tradition now becoming written.

References

Bartsch, H. W. (ed.) (1961). *Kerygma and Myth: Rudolf Bultmann and Five Critics. A Theological Debate.* New York: Harper Torchbooks.

Bermant, G. and Davidson, J. M. (1974). *Biological bases of sexual behavior.* New York: Harper and Row.

Bermant, G. (2005). *Seeing what is already there.* New York: American Buddhist Study Center.

Bermant, G. (2015). Already But Not Yet: Calling and Called in Religious Time. In D. B. Yaden, T. D. McCall, and J. H. Ellens (Eds.), *Being Called: Scientific, Secular, and Sacred Perspectives* (pp. 243–260). New York: Praeger.

Bermant, G. (2017a). Introduction to the Special Section on Subjectivity in Shin Buddhism. *Pacific World*, 19, 1–17.

Bermant, G. (2017b). The Nature and Importance of Subjectivity in Shin Buddhism. *Pacific World*, 19, 31–52.

Bogomilsky, M. (n.d.), Questions and Answers on the First-Fruits. From the Sichos in English Collection. *Chabad*. Available at: https://www.chabad.org/library/article_cdo/aid/2836645/jewish/The-First-Fruits.htm

Bultmann, R. (2007). *Theology of the New Testament* (K. Grobel, Trans.). Baylor University Press. (Original work published 1948.)

Bultmann, R. (1961a). New Testament and Mythology. In H. W. Bartsch (Ed.), *Kerygma and Myth: Rudolf Bultmann and Five Critics. A Theological Debate*. New York: Harper Torchbooks (pp. 1–44).

Bultmann, R. (1961b). A Reply to the Theses of J. Schniewind. In H. W. Bartsch (Ed.), *Kerygma and Myth: Rudolf Bultmann and Five Critics. A Theological Debate*. New York: Harper Torchbooks (pp. 102–123).

Capps, J. (2023). The Pragmatic Theory of Truth. In *The Stanford Encyclopedia of Philosophy*. (Original entry published 2019.) Available at: https://plato.stanford.edu/

Catechism of the Catholic Church. (1997). *Catechism of the Catholic Church*, 633–658. Vatican City: Libreria Editrice Vaticana.

Coyne, J. A. (2015). *Faith vs. Fact: Why Science and Religion are Incompatible*. New York: Viking.

Dawkins, R. (2006). *The God Delusion*. New York: Bantam Press.

Dennett, D. (2006). *Breaking the Spell: Religion as a Natural Phenomenon*. New York: Viking.

Ensign-George, B. (2021). What Presbyterians Believe About the Resurrection. *Presbyterian Mission Agency*, March 5. Available at: https://centernet.pcusa.org/story/pt-0321-wpb/

Farrow, D. (1999). *Ascencion and Ecclesia: On the Significance of the Doctrine of the Ascencion for Ecclesiology and Christian Cosmology*. Grand Rapids, MI: Eerdmans.

Gottlieb, M. (2023). A Jewish Theology of Resurrection. *First Things*, 337, November, 45–51.

Harris, S. (2006). *Letter to a Christian Nation*. New York: Knopf.

Harder, C. (n.d.). Why Do Lutherans Believe in the Resurrection of the Body? *Lutherans Restoring Creation*. Available at: https://lutheransrestoringcreation.org/why-do-lutherans-believe-in-the-resurrection-of-the-body/

Hitchens, C. (2007). *God Is Not Great*. New York: Twelve Books.

Hitchens, C., Dawkins, R., Harris, S., and Dennett, D. (2019). *The Four Horsemen: The Conversation that Sparked an Atheist Revolution*. New York: Random House.

Inagaki, H. and Stewart, H. (1994). *The Three Pure Land Sutras: A Study and Translation from Chinese*. Kyoto: Nagata Bunshodo.

James, W. (1902). *The Varieties of Religious Experience: A Study in Human Nature*. New York: Longmans, Green & Co.

Jastrow, M. and Friedländer, M. (n.d.). BIKKURIM "First-Fruits." *The Jewish Encyclopedia*. Available at: https://jewishencyclopedia.com/articles/3294-bikkurim

Keathley, J. H.III. (2004). Soteriology – the Doctrine of Salvation. *Bible.org*, May 17. Available at: https://bible.org/article/soteriology-doctrine-salvation

Lapide, P. (2002). *The Resurrection of Jesus: A Jewish Perspective*, trans. Wilhelm C. LinssEugene, OR: Augsburg.

Lohmeyer, E. (1961). The Right Interpretation of the Mythological. In H. W. Bartsch (Ed.), *Kerygma and Myth: Rudolf Bultmann and Five Critics. A Theological Debate*. New York: Harper Torchbooks (pp. 124–137).

Marshall, R. (n.d.). What Did Jesus Do for 40 Days after the Resurrection? *The Christian Broadcasting Network*. Available at: https://www2.cbn.com/article/salvation/what-did-jesus-do-40-days-after-resurrection

Moore, D. D. (1994). *To the Golden Cities: Pursuing the American Jewish Dream in Miami and L.A*. Cambridge, MA: Harvard University Press.

Mormon Wiki (n.d.) Mormon Beliefs: Resurrection. *Mormon Wiki*. Available at: https://www.mormonwiki.com/Mormon_Beliefs:_Resurrection

Orthodox Wiki. (2013). Resurrection. *Orthodox Wiki*, August 21. Available at: https://orthodoxwiki.org/index.php?title=Resurrection&oldid=116844

Schniewind, J. (1961). A Reply to Bultmann: Theses on the Emancipation of the Kerygma from Mythology. In H. W. Bartsch (Ed.) *Kerygma and Myth: Rudolf Bultmann and Five Critics. A Theological Debate*. New York: Harper Torchbooks (pp. 45–101).

Schumann, F. (1961). *Can the Event of Jesus Christ Be Demythologized?* In H. W. Bartsch (Ed.), *Kerygma and Myth: Rudolf Bultmann and Five Critics. A Theological Debate*. New York: Harper Torchbooks (pp. 175–190).

Sipress, D. (2013). God Entertains Prayers from Earth [Cartoon]. *New Yorker*, 89(3) March 4.

Swinburne, R. (2016). *The Coherence of Theism* (2nd edition). Oxford: Oxford University Press. (Original work published 1977.)

Thielicke, H. (1961). The Restatement of New Testament Mythology. In H. W. Bartsch (Ed.), *Kerygma and Myth: Rudolf Bultmann and Five Critics. A Theological Debate*. New York: Harper Torchbooks (pp. 138–174).

Weisman, J. (2023). Is Anti-Zionism Antisemitism, By Definition? The Question Roils the National Discourse. *New York Times*, December 12, A1, col. 5.

White, T. (n.d.). Seven Reasons to Believe in the Bodily Resurrection of Jesus Christ. *Leipers Fork Church of Christ*. Available at: https://www.leipersforkchurchofchrist.com/jesus-bodily-resurrection

Young, J. O. (2018). The Coherence Theory of Truth. In *The Stanford Encyclopedia of Philosophy*. (Original entry published 1996.) Available at: https://plato.stanford.edu/

Chapter 9

Emergent Phenomena and Spiritual Transformation

A Psychological and Autoethnographic Exploration

Vanessa Cha

At its core, this essay is a meditation on the question of what to make of spiritual experiences. Can some experiences be so extreme that they are inherently pathological, or can even seemingly extreme experiences be contained and channeled toward spiritual growth? These questions do not have easy answers, and I do not claim to hold them. Rather, this chapter represents the beginning of my inquiry, shaped by both my academic background and personal observations that largely emerged during my undergraduate years.

This chapter grows out of the idea that unusual phenomena that might, in isolation, be interpreted as psychiatric symptoms, can potentially be described by a different path when offered containment within a more spiritual framework. These unexpected experiences can include: a deep sense of interconnectedness between seemingly unconnected events, people, memories, and sensations; sudden overwhelming sorrow and joy, sometimes simultaneously; odd bodily sensations; visions; and more. They can also include despair, a breakdown in how one makes meaning, relationship crises, and even a sense that one is going "crazy." In particular, this examination will highlight how mindfulness and meditative practices can, unto themselves, evoke or exacerbate such emergent phenomena which call for the support and structure of spiritual direction, mentoring, or an intentional community of practitioners. As I describe in the latter portion of this chapter, these experiences are common enough to demand a reassessment of the casual recommendation of mindfulness and meditative technologies without ongoing support. Therefore, I offer this chapter with its cataloging of research initiatives to support mental health professionals and spiritual mentors alike.

Throughout this journey, I have come to appreciate that reality extends far beyond what the naked eye perceives—something science has long confirmed in its own way. What we see is not necessarily all there is, but rather a reflection of what our biology and psychology allow us to perceive.

This limitation in perception extends beyond the physical world to how we understand and categorize human behavior. Through my studies and personal observations, I've noticed a common tendency—particularly in Western frameworks—to categorize behavior and perceived differences in ways that can

DOI: 10.4324/9781003742852-9

inadvertently put people in boxes, leading to the pathologization of those who think or perceive differently from dominant socio-cultural norms. In some cases, this categorization can be beneficial and empowering for the individual; in others, it may risk doing more harm than good.

Culture, developmental appropriateness, and pathology—to name a few factors—become difficult to weigh when attempting to judge someone else's subjective experiences. In psychology, we are apt to use words such as reality testing, self-concept, ego integrity, and theory of mind to assess someone's ability to make sense of their surroundings, their "reality," and their capacity to make distinctions between themselves and the Other.[1] This is a part of the human condition that represents a fundamental evolutionary achievement. For if, as *Homo sapiens*, we can't make these subject/object distinctions, or distinguish between us and the Other, then we likely would not have survived as a species. In other words, we'd be eaten by a hungry sabretooth tiger or starve to death as we wouldn't be able to relate to our environment and our community in a meaningful way. Today, these differentiations persist—not just for survival but as a way to create order, shared meaning, and understanding. We categorize: male or female, White or Black, and draw neat, tidy lines on a map to separate us from them. These distinctions help us orient ourselves in the world, yet they come at a cost—reducing our ability to perceive nuance. This compromise enables us to assert a type of utilitarian truth, but too often at the expense of the kind of truth born through experience—that is, wisdom.

Science thrives through clarity of definitions. We have to find a common language in order to facilitate progress. The progression is always towards some truth or knowing—which is, at its highest level in materialist science, the cause-effect relationship; however, to statistically validate or prove such relationships exist often comes at a cost. Independent variables are assessed in isolation to determine their effects on the dependent outcome variable of interest; yet human experience does not unfold in a petri dish or a randomized control trial.

This tension between established categories and lived complexity is also echoed in the philosophy of science and Buddhism. The philosopher of science, Thomas Kuhn (2012 [1962]), proposes that scientific knowledge does not progress linearly, but rather through a series of revolutions. This paradigm shift occurs when a new anomaly—in this case emergent phenomena—threatens the current understanding of science—that is pathology—and a crisis emerges in which the old existing framework fails to be adopted to explain such an anomaly. This causes a radical shift to form a new paradigm that better explains this anomaly and a new norm is established.

From a Buddhist perspective, science may be understood as operating within the realm of relative reality or relative truth, the realm of conceptual distinctions such as right versus wrong, or pathology versus emergent phenomena. While science excels at discerning objective facts and statistically valid measures, it often falls short in capturing the truth of one's lived experience, as a test cannot fully grasp the complex heterogeneous mixture of phenomena that shape our lived reality. Buddhism contends that the absolute reality or absolute truth is beyond concept and subject–object distinctions. Yet, in another classically paradoxical Buddhist perspective, the absolute truth and the relative truth are both one and the same (Rinpoche, 2015). The relative truth may be thought of as a mere reflection of the absolute truth in our subjective, objective reality. Just as the reflection of the moon in the water is not a perfect image, neither is the relative truth, yet it may be the closest we can get to touching the moon. The discernment of one's truth ultimately rests in the individual's interpretation of their subjective experiences—an interpretation that can be guided with the support of spiritual directors, clinicians, and therapists through different frameworks.

The following pages are a synthesis of anecdotal information; information drawn from religious ideologies and theories; research in the field of existentialism; ideas from Jung, object-relations, transpersonal psychology, and clinical psychology; and neuroscientific findings—all collated in an attempt to answer one question: what differentiates pathological distortions of reality and those that may be spiritually transformative?

A Brief Biographical Note

I was born in Northern Alberta, Canada, to a Korean immigrant father and a Caucasian Canadian mother. Though raised within Christian traditions, I was not immersed in formal religious life. Still, from an early age, I was preoccupied with existential questions—"Why am I here? What is my purpose?"—and eventually turned toward Buddhism and other esoteric practices in search of deeper answers.

In Search of Absolute Truth: A Personal Awakening

The Buddha was thrust into his journey by the four sights: death, old age, sickness, and a monk. For me, it was a painful betrayal at the age of 20. That rupture led me to question the very framework of my reality, in which I began searching for some "Ultimate Truth." But instead of answers, I encountered a shift in perspective: that freedom came not from grasping for some fixed or relative truth, but in releasing the need for certainty altogether. I let go of my attachment to some singular, ultimate understanding and began to embrace the subjectivity and fluidity of one's experience. I realized that we may not be able to fully grasp another's absolute truth, just as we often struggle to grasp our own. What we perceive as absolute may itself evolve as we deepen our awareness and expand our consciousness. In this way, truth is not fixed but emergent—unfolding alongside our growth, our healing, and our capacity to perceive more clearly.

This cognitive shift also catalyzed an energetic one: what once felt like a void in my chest became a radiant, embodied presence—what I came to understand as divine love. This was the first mystical experience I had encountered since childhood, and it awakened in me a renewed sense of purpose, beginning to answer the questions I had carried for so long. In the years that followed, I became increasingly attuned to the subtle sensations of my body and energy. This marked the beginning of a different kind of listening and a deeper unveiling of my absolute truth—one that would continue to unfold through somatic experiences, energetic clearings, and eventually, the practice of Reiki. I later came to realize my experiences were not unique but echoed across various religious, philosophical, and psychological frameworks.[2]

These experiences and insights also led me to reorient my academic path. While working as a primary care medical assistant, I witnessed first-hand the true healing powers of empathy and compassionate listening, which inspired me to change my major to psychology. It was here, in the spring semester of my third year, that I found myself in a clinical psychology class led by Aaron B. Daniels. Under his mentorship, I began to bridge my personal awakening with academic inquiry—joining a Psychological Humanities Workgroup, guiding meditations at a university spiritual life center, and helping organize a Mindfulness Body-Mind Forum at an international conference. During this time, I also joined the Harvard Meditation Research Program and the Northeastern EPIC Brain Lab, where I explored the questions of what to make of emergent phenomena and where—and if—we should draw the line between spiritual emergence and pathology. It has been a journey marked by inquiry, reflection, and transformation.

As I continued deepening into both psychological study and somatic expression, I became increasingly aware of how these transformations weren't only mental or spiritual—they were deeply physical. This led me to consider how our bodies themselves might participate in the unfolding truth, healing, and spiritual insight.

Somatic Phenomenology

Our mind, body, and spirit are deeply interconnected, something that Eastern philosophies and ancient healing practices have long understood. The scientific community has further validated this mind–body connection showing a complex interplay between our gut microbiome, our neuroendocrine systems, and the central nervous system, which has been shown to regulate cognition, behavior, mood, and psychiatric disorders (Adzic et al., 2015; Dicks, 2024; Peng et al., 2025). However, the scientific understanding of spirit is still in its infancy.

We all have experienced aspects of our emotions somatically, whether that be stress manifesting itself as tension headaches, tightness in the jaw and shoulders, or the feeling of our heart racing and palms sweating as our sympathetic nervous system kicks in and we experience a rush of noradrenaline and adrenaline. Others, including myself, have suffered from a range of gastrointestinal difficulties such as "chronic abdominal pain" or irritable bowel syndrome (IBS) which has been linked to somatic manifestations of anxiety and trauma (Afari et al., 2014; Jacobs and Whitehead, 2014; Popa and Dumitrascu, 2015). The remedy for my pain eventually came when my parents took me to see an acupuncturist—an experience that would later shape my understanding of the intricate connection between mind and body. As I have become more attuned to the subtleties of my own experiences, it has become increasingly clear to me that my body was not just passively responding to my emotions and the emotions of others but was holding onto them. Trauma, stress, and anxiety are not just psychological experiences—they are physical realities imprinted in our muscles, nervous system, and even gut, that may manifest themselves as tensions or pain in the body.

In Eastern medicine, particularly acupuncture and the systems of Classical and Traditional Chinese Medicine, these physical manifestations are recognized as disruptions in *Qi*—the body's energy flow. Thus, treatments work to restore this balance of flow. Research supports the efficacy of acupuncture in reducing symptoms of IBS and alleviating anxiety (Wang et al., 2022). While our minds may not be consciously aware of it, our bodies may act as the gatekeepers to our unconscious, storing and expressing what the mind suppresses. In this way, a physical symptom may well force us to pay attention; but too often we end up paying attention to the symptom and not the system giving rise to it.

If my personal awakening brought me closer to divine love, it also opened a door to experiencing other somatic sensations—many for which I had no conceptual framework at the time. Some of these somatic sensations arose spontaneously, during meditative practice and during eye movement desensitization and reprocessing (EMDR) therapy. While some somatic sensations I have been able to label and integrate through therapy relatively easily, there have been other sensations I have experienced that transcend the framework of most modern-day psychologists and clinicians. I have been lucky to have found containment and a framework for interpreting such somatic phenomena through a less conventional healing modality—energy healing, which attempts to restore the body's energy flow. I have found that while EMDR therapy can intensify somatic sensations, energy healing has been incredibly effective in releasing residual energy, stressors, and even trauma that may have been processed mentally but remains stored in the body.

All energy healing modalities are thought to work with the life force or life energy. This life force has been given many names across cultures: *Chi* or *Qi* in Chinese, *Prana* in Sanskrit, and *Ti* or *Ki* in Hawaiian or Kanji (Rand, 2019, p. 3). In contemporary scientific literature, it is often referred to as the biofield, defined as "the energy and materials that surround and permeate the human body" (Trivedi et al., 2024, p. 1). This life force flows around us in our aura and within the physical body through pathways known as chakras, meridians, or *nadis* (Rand, 2019, p. 8).

One popular modality of energy healing is Reiki, a stress reduction and relaxation technique originating in Japan in which a practitioner acts as a conduit to channel universal energy that promotes healing for the client.[3]

While the mechanisms of such practices remain largely debated in the scientific community, several randomized controlled trials have shown that energy healing, specifically Reiki, is an effective complementary therapy in pain management and mental illnesses such as anxiety, and improving quality of life for those with chronic illness and cancer (Liu et al., 2025; McManus, 2017; Morero et al., 2021; Thrane and Cohen, 2014; Trivedi et al., 2024). This suggests that energy healing practices exceed the placebo effect. In addition to the ongoing research, Reiki is becoming increasingly offered as a complementary therapy in integrative medicine centers and oncology units such as Cleveland Clinic, Beth Israel Deaconess Medical Center, and Memorial Sloan Kettering.

During these energy clearings I, like many others with whom I've spoken, often experience a current of energy coursing through my body, shifting tensions, body twitches, cooling and warming sensations, and other residual energies as they are released. At times, this process triggers a cathartic release, manifesting as deep, uncontrollable crying and intense bodily shaking. Such unusual somatic experiences may also arise during meditation, something I would soon encounter in my own research.

Exploring the Prevalence of Emergent Phenomena

It was the winter of 2023 when I began working as a research assistant at the Harvard Meditation Research Program. This lab, led by Matthew Sacchett, focuses on advancing the scientific understanding of meditation phenomena. During my time at the Harvard Meditation Research Program, I worked on a research project led by Malcolm Wright, which focused on analyzing emergent phenomena (EP)—a type of altered state of consciousness, defined as "sudden unusual mental or somatic experiences often interpreted as spiritual, mystical, energetic, or magical in nature" (Wright et al., 2024, p. 2).

I entered the meditation research space completely unaware of the vast depths of human phenomena I was about to join the team in exploring. I had initially thought of meditation as something only beneficial that could do no harm. With the huge surge in the wellness and meditation market, meditation and mindfulness practices have found their way into schools from elementary level all the way up to college (Mikhail, 2024). In the workplace, it is used to enhance focus, performance, and productivity. Meditation has also become incorporated into different therapeutic techniques, most commonly used as a method for reducing stress and anxiety. These therapeutic approaches include mindfulness-based stress reduction, acceptance and commitment therapy, dialectical behavior therapy, and many others. In the past decade, more research has been published that shows the clinical benefits of meditation, even for treating symptoms of schizophrenia and depression (Bauer et al.,

2020; Hofmann et al., 2010; Sabe et al., 2019; Zhang et al., 2023). Yet, I have found through my work at the Harvard Meditation Research Program that meditation can begin to unravel our psyche, allowing unconscious material to bubble up into our consciousness, resulting in experiences that can at times be destabilizing. Such transient distress as a result of meditation is seen at a similar rate to other psychological interventions (Britton et al., 2021).

Commercialized mindfulness and meditation programs and apps promise the benefit of producing and enhancing well-being without any labeled side effects. Yet, as Wright et al. (2024) noted, mindfulness practices can also produce altered states of consciousness that can trigger changes in sense of self and worldview. These transformative experiences are often associated with EP I mentioned at the outset of this chapter. EP are not restricted to a meditative setting but may arise spontaneously or be preceded by a psychological trigger. Wright et al. (2025, p. 2) clarify that EP is

> similar to but somewhat broader in scope than altered states of consciousness because they (a) do not assume a baseline against which alteration occurs; (b) often manifest as a fluid or evolving experience rather than being a rigid, stable state; and (c) may include somatic and mental elements and even the cessation of consciousness altogether.

In the past, these EPs have been referred to as spiritual emergencies or transpersonal crises, terms first introduced by Grof and Grof (1989). In the meditation literature, authors often refer to these events as "unpleasant," "unwanted," "adverse," and challenging (cf., Schlosser et al., 2019; Cebolla et al., 2017; Shapiro, 1992; Lomas et al., 2015). However, while such phenomena can be challenging, they may also be seen by some individuals as normal or positive depending on the type of experience or cultural context in which it arises (Cebolla et al., 2017; Grof and Grof, 2017). The rise in popularity of spiritual disciplines such as meditation in the West—and the emergent phenomena that can arise with them—necessitate further research into this field of study.

Jared Lindahl and Willoughby Britton are among the leaders in such meditation research. Their qualitative studies on the Varieties of Contemplative Experience (VCE) have explored the range of meditative experiences based on interviews from more than 30 Buddhist teachers and 60 Buddhist practitioners from Theravada, Zen, and Tibetan traditions. From this VCE collection, Lindahl et al. (2017) identified 59 categories of meditation-related effects and grouped them into seven phenomenological domains: cognition, perception, emotion, physical sensations, behavior, sense of self, and social aspects. They found that 73% of practitioners reported experiences in six or more domains. Some of the most common phenomenologies reported were: fear, anxiety, panic, or paranoia (82%); changes in motivation or goal (78%); positive affect (75%); sleep changes (62%); depression, dysphoria, or grief (57%); changes in self-other or self-world boundaries (53%); social impairment (50%); and somatic energy (63%). This somatic energy was reported as an electricity-like "voltage" or "currents" running through the body that were sometimes associated with the release of pressure or tension that can be accompanied with involuntary movements. When I read these descriptions—and the jaw-dropping percentages of those having these experiences—I couldn't help but see that this somatic energy explained by the researchers was not unlike what I've encountered during mediation—and in the tension releases I've experienced during energetic clearing.

A more recent study by Britton, Lindal, and colleagues highlighted that such meditation-related side effects (MRSE) occur even in mindfulness-based programs. Their findings of a representative sample of 96 Americans with affective disturbances found that 83% reported experiencing at least one MRSE, with the majority reporting multiple MRSEs (Britton et al., 2021).

The study by Wright et al. (2024) analyzed the prevalence of emergent phenomena on a much larger scale, including those outside of the meditation context, by generating a representative population survey completed by 3,135 UK and US-based participants.

Wright et al. (2024) found that 26% of participants, while not on mind-altering substances, reported supernatural or miraculous events, with the most common reports being forms of precognitive knowledge (10%); visions of other beings such as angels, demons, spirits, ghosts, or djinni (7%); knowledge of distant events (6%); and knowledge of others' thoughts (6%). Another question assessing emergent phenomena found that 45% of participants reported experiencing non-pharmacologically induced sudden unusual mental events at least once in their lives. These included symptoms of derealization (17%); a strong sense of oneness with the world or with God (15%); ecstatic thrills (15%); vivid perceptions (11%); changes in perceived size (10%); bodily heat or electricity (9%); and out-of-body experiences (8%). Wright's team then assessed the valence to well-being in which these events were perceived. Based on their analysis, Wright et al. contended that this relationship is not determinative. That is, while positively perceived events are more likely to lead to positive changes to well-being, negatively perceived events could also lead to positive changes to well-being. This unclear relationship may reflect the complex psychological process of integration, where adaptation and meaning-making may mediate or moderate the eventual effect on well-being (Wright et al., 2024). In a meditation context, how one's experience is appraised may be in part due to the practitioners having different conceptual frameworks or worldviews (Lindahl et al., 2017).

Regarding the type of negative experiences, most reported "Feelings of misery, sadness, or disgust with [their] life" and "A disturbing sense that the world is nothing but a dream or cartoon" (Wright et al., 2024, p. 7). Wright et al. also found that 19.1% of participants reported varying degrees of suffering, with 57% of individuals who experienced moderate to life-threatening levels reporting a mental health diagnosis. While not entirely synonymous to

Wright et al.'s construct of "suffering," Britton et al. (2021) found that 58% of their patients with affective disorders in their meditation study reported their adverse experience as unpleasant at the time it occurred (i.e., negatively valenced), and 37% reported them as still unpleasant in hindsight (i.e., negative impact). In addition, 29.5% experienced lasting bad effects from meditation, with durations lasting from one day to five or more months. This suggests that individuals with existing mental illness may be more susceptible to EP-related distress. At the same time, such distress may closely resemble symptoms of psychopathology and is often diagnosed as such within clinical settings.

Another striking finding from Wright et al.'s (2024) study was that 63% of those who experienced suffering did not seek help and only 47% had heard of the risk of unpleasant experiences that could arise from spiritual or meditative practice. Wright et al. contended that this may be due to individuals fearing that clinicians will not understand their experiences or subjects may just have overall uncertainty about where to seek help. This reluctance for individuals to reach out to clinicians makes sense as many individuals may fear their mystical or spiritual experiences may be misunderstood and pathologized. Myself along with others whom I have met have been faced with this fear, but I have been fortunate enough to have found individuals (e.g., mentors, teachers, body workers, and psychotherapists) who have understood, validated, and provided containment for my experiences.

The implications of Wright et al.'s (2024) work stretch well beyond their sample of meditators into the broader population, whose endorsed experiences of spirituality, transcendence, or the supernatural challenge our understanding of reality. We hear of spiritual mediums and shamans who can communicate with spirits and the dead. Many cultures and individuals believe that there is something beyond ourselves, a connection to the other world(s) or the divine; yet others simply refuse to believe that in which they cannot see, and pathologize such experiences. It is very likely that in certain instances, individuals who present themselves as being "spiritually gifted" may be charlatans or psychologically ill or both. Nevertheless, some individuals may demonstrate perceptual abilities that challenge the dimensional realms we call reality—abilities that might better be measured and described in empirical qualitative ways. It may very well be that we all possess such abilities within ourselves, such emergent phenomena which may arise spontaneously or be uncovered through meditative practices or other esoteric rituals. This is evident given the fact that 26% and 45% of Wright et al.'s (2024) subjects experienced supernatural or miraculous events or emergent phenomena, respectively. Such findings underscore the importance of being able to differentiate between pathology and spiritual phenomena. This is not just a minor subset of people who are having these experiences. Individuals in our Westernized culture are having mystical and bizarre experiences that cannot be explained by science without resorting to unnuanced and habitual pathologization. Again, we must accept the possibility that while some experiences may be pathological in nature and demand psychiatric attention, others may be something entirely different.

The urgent question is clear: how can we know? How can we discern between those who need mindfulness, meditation, and/or spiritual support and those who demand urgent mental health interventions? Diagnoses of pathology are complex and difficult. Psycho- and physical pathology aren't that different and can at times, if not always, be one and the same, as the fields of neurology, neuropsychiatry, and neuropsychology testify. Just as there are numerous different causes as to why someone has a headache or numerous different diseases and viruses that cause similar symptoms, the etiology of an individual's mental state differs, although the symptoms at first glance may appear the same. Emergent phenomena are not very easy to diagnose or differentiate since the symptoms could stem from anywhere (e.g., past trauma, clinical issues, or a recent event). Consider a theoretical clinical example: John just returned from a long retreat and is feeling jittery, but he also stopped drinking coffee after the retreat. Is the cause of Johns's jitters a symptom of emergent phenomena that has arisen from the retreat or from the fact that John is in withdrawal from caffeine? There are many factors that could be intertwined that are difficult to parse out and they are not necessarily mutually exclusive. For example, John's jitters may be attributed to emergent phenomena arising from the retreat, which could be further exacerbated by his decision to stop drinking coffee.

It is up to us, the clinicians, psychotherapists, companions, and spiritual practitioners, to be compassionate detectives in this arising phenomenology, to use our acquired knowledge and examination skills, but not to forget that the current frontiers of science cannot explain everything.

What Are the "Risk" Factors?

The current literature suggests that the risk of experiencing emergent phenomena (EP) is shaped by a complex interplay of personal, contextual, and practice-related variables. Lindahl et al.'s (2017) work offers an intimate window into the lives of meditators who found themselves overwhelmed by experiences that felt spiritual, psychological, or both. The work I conducted alongside my supervisor, Malcolm Wright (Wright et al., 2025) builds on that picture, showing that these patterns are not isolated—many of the same risk and protective factors appear across a much larger and more diverse group of people. For instance, both studies suggest that an individual's personal history may shape their likelihood of encountering such experiences.

Lindahl et al. (2017) emphasized that the individual's medical, psychological, and trauma history, as well as personality and temperament, must be considered. The supportiveness of early-life relationships can influence both personality traits and the likelihood of psychiatric or trauma-related vulnerability. Traumatic experiences, in particular, may be reactivated during meditation, unveiling painful emotions or repressed memories and potentially leading to somatic manifestations and distress (Goldberg et al., 2022; Miller, 1993). Similarly, our study found that history of a mental illness, a traumatic or spiritually powerful childbirth experience, and lower self-perceived adjustment increased one's risk of experiencing EP. These factors were also shown to increase one's risk of subsequent suffering following EP, with one difference: lower self-perceived mental health replaced self-perceived adjustment.

Not surprisingly, personal relationships and connections within the meditation community are important factors in how individuals interpret and integrate their experiences (Lindahl et al., 2017). The role of the teacher was particularly influential—when teachers were present, supportive, and empathetic, they helped create a sense of safety and fostered beneficial outcomes. In contrast, a lack of guidance or a mismatch in values between teacher and student increased the likelihood of negative meditation effects or emergent phenomena. Lindahl et al. also emphasized the significance of compatibility between the practitioner's experiences and their teacher's worldview, goals, and cultural framework. A shared sociocultural context could serve as a remedy, offering grounding and validation. But when there was a mismatch—between cultural backgrounds, social customs, or interpretive frameworks—the sociocultural context itself could become a risk factor.

We can see how these dynamics may extend beyond meditation. Whether in therapy, medicine, or spiritual direction, the degree of trust, cultural sensitivity, and mutual understanding between patient and guide deeply shapes whether an individual feels safe enough to process and integrate profound or destabilizing experiences.

In a similar manner, religiosity may make individuals less susceptible to experiencing unpleasant meditation-related experiences, both through the protective effect of a strong sense of community and in viewing such phenomena as sacred (Castillo, 1990; Schlosser et al., 2019). In traditions like Buddhism, these "unusual" or "bizarre" experiences are sometimes viewed as potential distractions or temptations that may obstruct one's progress toward enlightenment if clung to. However, they are also recognized as normal and expected byproducts of intense meditative practice—especially during serious vipassana practice (Lindahl et al., 2019).

Interestingly, our population-level study found no significant association between religiosity and either the occurrence of EP or subsequent suffering. However, we did find that individuals who self-identified as less spiritual were more likely to experience EP, but less likely to suffer afterward.

This finding suggests a more nuanced relationship: spirituality, like religiosity, may act as a buffer against experiencing EP, perhaps through shared meaning-making and social support. Yet, for those who do experience EP, higher levels of spirituality may paradoxically increase the risk of suffering. This may be especially prevalent if the experience destabilizes or contradicts one's spiritual worldview. In such cases, the dissonance between expectation and reality may lead to fragility or distress within the spiritual framework, disrupting the very sense of coherence that spirituality typically provides.

These complexities raise important questions about how spiritual and psychological frameworks interact, especially as meditative practices become increasingly secularized and adapted for therapeutic use. This points to a growing concern in the secularization process. While this at large is beneficial and makes such modalities more accessible, we must air caution as to not to strip the practice entirely from its roots. Clinicians, therapist spiritual directors, and wellness facilitators must be aware of the cultural context from which such practices emerge. Meditation's original purpose was not to treat psychopathology as we know it today but rather to reach nirvana, spiritual freedom, and end suffering (*dukkha*). Buddhist philosophy understands suffering as a fundamental aspect of human experience, arising from attachment and ignorance. In this sense, mental distress—including what might be labeled as psychopathology—can be seen as a form of suffering, though the frameworks for understanding and addressing it differ. Thus, as mental health professionals and spiritual mentors in a globalized, multicultural world, we must look beyond the DSM and Westernized views of psychopathology, broadening our understanding of mental distress as it is conceptualized across different cultures and spiritual traditions.

This cultural nuance becomes even more relevant when considering how demographic factors, such as ethnicity and age, might influence one's experience of EP. In our study (Wright et al., 2025), we found that identifying as Asian and being older in age decreased one's likelihood of experiencing EP. Older age also decreased the likelihood of suffering; however, this finding may be due to the recent rise in mindfulness and meditation practices among younger individuals, who may thus have more exposure to EP.

Conversely, identifying as an "other" ethnicity (i.e. non-White or non-Asian) emerged as risk factors for experiencing both EP and subsequent suffering. While our data cannot explain *why* these patterns emerged, it's important to consider the broader sociocultural context. Given that the population data comes from UK and US participants, it may reflect the ways in which racialized minority groups often face greater marginalization, cumulative stress, or trauma exposure—factors that may sensitize individuals and make them more susceptible to EP. Furthermore, the increased likelihood of suffering among these groups may be partly due to a mismatch between their cultural background and the predominantly Western secular or East Asian Buddhist and Hindu paradigms that dominate many meditation and yoga spaces. These paradigms may not offer interpretive tools, language, or community that feel relevant or safe for those from other cultural or spiritual backgrounds.

Another important yet unsurprising factor is healthy behaviors. Lindahl et al. (2017) found practitioners reported healthy behaviors as remedies to the distress of EP when present or in balance and as potential risk factors when absent or out of balance. Just think of a time when you were overworked, overstressed, not getting proper sleep and taking care of your mental and physical health. How were you functioning? This puts us at risk for a multitude of both physical and mental ailments. Although we may think of meditation as a wellness behavior exclusively, its power does not render it immune to such contextual factors.

Notably, our study (Wright et al., 2025) found that it is not the religious or spiritual practices (i.e., Christianity or Buddhism) per se, but rather the practice technique—such as loving-kindness meditation, mindfulness of the body, breath- or movement-based practices, contemplation of mysteries, dwelling in unity with God or the World, and other specific meditative or spiritual practices that were not listed on the survey—that predicted the likelihood of experiencing EP.

A separate large-scale survey (Schlosser et al., 2019) further clarified this by comparing deconstructive and non-deconstructive (attentional) types of meditation. Deconstructive practices—aimed at dissolving ordinary assumptions about self, reality, and time (e.g., *vispanna* [insight] and *shikantaza* ["just sitting"])—were associated with a 65% higher likelihood of unpleasant meditation-related experiences compared to those who only engaged in non-deconstructive (attentional) practices. Such attentional practices are designed to stabilize and focus attention, such as mindfulness of breathing, mindfulness of the body, and Jhana practices.[4]

The cumulation of these findings may suggest that deconstructive practices may be more disorienting and distressing compared to attention-based practices. However, this does not mean they do not elicit EP; rather, the EP they produce may be appraised more positively or be less likely to result in distress or suffering. This interpretation aligns with our findings (Wright et al., 2025) that all practice techniques, aside from contemplation of mysteries, did not increase one's likelihood of experiencing subsequent suffering. Contemplation of mysteries may function similarly to deconstructive practices in that they challenge conventional understandings of self and reality. This may further explain why our findings found it associated with increased likelihood of subsequent suffering (Wright et al., 2025).

Interestingly, prayer was found to be protective, decreasing the likelihood of EP. This suggests that substituting prayer for mindfulness-based practices may reduce EP occurrence.

We found that spiritual or meditative practice outside retreat settings, a measure of the total dose of practice in non-supervised settings, increased ones risk of experiencing EP and subsequent suffering (Wright et al., 2025). This finding is consistent with previous research suggesting that more extensive practice and individual unsupervised practice outside formal retreats may increase one's likelihood of experiencing meditation-related unusual or adverse effects (Britton et al., 2021; Cebolla et al., 2017; Goldberg et al., 2022). However, other studies have found that retreat settings themselves can increase the risk of experiencing EP (Dyga and Stupak, 2015; Schlosser et al., 2019). This may be due to the intensive and often silent nature of certain retreats, which frequently emphasize deconstructive practices such as *vipassana* and typically offer minimal interpersonal interaction or psychological support. These findings reiterate the importance of containment through support, connection and guidance.

In Lindahl et al.'s (2017) study, practitioners in the study also cited recreational drug use as a risk factor for certain experiences. Yet, interestingly, prior drug-related experiences were also reported as helpful in negotiating certain types of destabilizing meditation-related experiences.

I have heard anecdotes in the academic and meditation community that explain how both psychedelics and meditation have the potential to tap into similar, if not the same altered states of consciousness. Consider this analogy: psychedelics are like taking the elevator up, you push the button, and there's no stopping or going back. Meditation, on the other hand, is like taking the stairs: it's slow and a lot more work, but you can stop climbing and turn back at any time. In other words, meditation tends to offer individuals much more control over their experiences. However, there may be instances even in meditation where an individual may lose control and the stairs may start moving in an escalator-like fashion, taking them on an unexpected journey.

Our study (Wright et al., 2025) found that the three largest risk factors for experiencing both EP and subsequent suffering included psychedelic use; attempting divine, occult, or magical practices; and contemplating mysteries in practice. Divine magical, or occult practices referred to intentional spiritual or metaphysical activities such as healing prayer, banishing, spirit contact, mind reading, clairvoyance, divination, astral travel, spell casting, and telekinesis. These practices may increase vulnerability to EP and subsequent suffering especially when used without adequate containment or support.

To return to the earlier metaphor: engaging in occult practices or contemplative inquiry into esoteric themes—especially when paired with meditation—may act as an accelerator in this process. For individuals already facing systemic stress or who lack supportive interpretive frameworks, these practices may heighten their susceptibility to EP and the risk of suffering that follows.

It is important to note that while our study (Wright et al., 2025) offers important insight into the influential factors associated with EP and subsequent suffering, much remains to be explored—particularly regarding how these factors interact. For example, the causality of our predictor variables is not always clear. We don't know, for instance, whether psychedelics were used before or after EP occurred, or which type of psychedelic was involved. Nor did we assess interactions between variables—such as whether certain practices amplify the effects of others. It is likely that some may be complementary—amplifying or modulating each other's effects.

In my own case, I have used the aforementioned mindfulness of the body techniques for about three years, gradually becoming more attuned and aware to subtle somatic sensations and energetic patterns—often experienced as tensions or tingling sensations. I have carried this awareness beyond my meditative practice and at times, I've found myself contemplating if a sensation I am experiencing is purely physical or if it carries emotional, spiritual, or intuitive significance. As I meditate on these sensations, I often feel a shift: the energy begins to move, sometimes leading to a vision in my mind's eye which I interpret as a symbolic representation of the somatic energies that are asking to be released. On several occasions, this has culminated in a cathartic cry and a complete dissolution of the somatic sensations. Consistent with the literature, while mindfulness, contemplation, and energy-sensing may appear benign in isolation, in combination, they form a synergistic process that appears to elicit and process emergent experiences.

This points to a broader question: how might different combinations of personal characteristics and practices shape not only the likelihood of experiencing EP, but also the type of EP—and how might these be distinguished from pathology? While the identified risk factors offer a starting point for distinguishing spiritual difficulties from psychotic disorders, the reality is often complex, as such factors do not necessarily exclude the possibility of pathology. In addition, the interaction of multiple variables—psychological, cultural, spiritual, and neurological—makes it difficult to arrive at definitive conclusions. Such nuance invites a deeper investigation into the boundaries between pathology, and EP. For instance, Lindhal et al.'s (2017) VCE study found that 47% of participants reported "delusional, irrational, or paranormal beliefs," 42% reported "hallucinations, visions, or illusions," and 17% reported "affective flattening or emotional detachment." These phenomena are commonly described as psychotic symptoms and associated with diagnoses such as schizophrenia or schizotypal personality disorder. Comparably, a narrative review by Sharma et al. (2019) assessed 19 studies with 28 cases of psychosis associated with meditation. Sharma et al. found that various types of meditation precipitated psychotic-like symptoms in which the cases' duration of psychosis ranged from a very brief episode to years. Out of the 28 cases, 14 cases were diagnosed with acute psychosis, seven with schizophrenia, three with mania and psychotic symptoms, and one with schizoaffective disorder. Similar to previous findings by Lindahl et al. (2017) and Wright et al., (2025), Sharma et al. (2019) noted that certain dispositions, like a history of mental illness, psychoactive substance abuse, stress, insomnia, and lack of food intake, could have influenced these states.

Meditation: A Double-Edged Sword

In this way, meditation is like a double-edged sword. While it can help alleviate symptoms of psychopathology, it may also cause or at least contribute to these symptoms. This paradox raises an important clinical question: how can we determine if meditation should be prescribed to alleviate symptoms of mental illness or avoided to prevent subsequent distress or adverse effects?

It may be that such risks are inherently unavoidable, but are not necessarily greater than those posed by other psychological intervention (Britton et al., 2021). However, just as ethical protocols are required for other treatments, it may be beneficial to provide individuals with a comprehensive understanding of the potential benefits and risks of the meditation or mindfulness practice they are about to undertake. This allows them to make an informed decision about whether they wish to embark on the journey.

At the same time, the combination of influential factors—such as mental health history, current stressors, and spiritual orientation— may provide useful guidance. Yet, it is often those with a history of mental illness who are referred to meditation-based interventions. Therefore, a better understanding on how meditation may trigger, modulate, or alleviate symptoms of mental illness could offer deeper insights into when and how it should be applied.

A specific regimen of meditation intervention in a clinical setting may be beneficial—particularly when practices are brief, guided, and offered with adequate support. Informal or unsupervised mindfulness practices may be more problematic, especially for individuals with serious mental illness, as these have been associated with lasting adverse effects such as hyperarousal and dissociation in patients with affective disorders (Britton et al., 2021).

Currently, meditation treatments for mental illness have utilized eight-week mindfulness meditation interventions (MMI), which typically include short, guided meditation focusing on the breath and a body scan. These practices fall under the umbrella of mindfulness of the body techniques, which, according to our study (Wright et al., 2025), may increase the likelihood of experiencing EP but are not significantly associated with subsequent suffering.

When conducted under guidance of a trained clinician—especially one culturally informed and prepared to support EP—MMIs may provide the containment needed to help individuals integrate challenging experiences safely. Additionally, MMIs have been shown to reduce levels of rumination, a common psychopathological feature in depression, anxiety, and psychosis (Dyga and Stupak, 2015; Reangsing et al., 2020; Schreiner and Malcolm, 2008). However, individuals with higher levels of rumination may also be more susceptible to experiencing emergent phenomena, as they may lack the ability to disengage their thinking patterns during meditation (Schlosser et al., 2019). So, while meditation may help disengage from ruminating thoughts, if one does not learn to control their rumination and continues to more advanced forms of meditation, they may be more likely to experience unusual mental phenomena as distressing.

Meditation can also help shift one's perspective on their mental illness from being integrated into one's identity to being separate from oneself (Dyga and Stupak, 2015; Schreiner and Malcolm, 2008). Conversely, overidentification with emergent phenomena may result in psychosis if individuals are unable to separate themselves from the experience (Dyga and Stupak, 2015). It seems we must train our minds to not over-identify and attach ourselves to the arising and passing of experiences. As Dharma teachings remind us, we must learn to "let go"—to witness without clinging. Attachment to any arising phenomena, whether pleasant or unpleasant, can be a source of suffering.

Pathology and Emergent Phenomena: A Journey Toward a Differential Diagnosis

While various Buddhist traditions share these core insights, they also have diverged in how they interpret emergent phenomena. For instance, Tibetan Buddhism may view certain states as untrustworthy hinderances to insight in one context and as signs of progress in another (Lindahl et al., 2017). This again brings us back to the central question—do these symptoms truly align with the criteria for a mental illness as defined by the DSM and our Westernized social constructs, or can there be other explanations? What differentiates a spiritual experience from a pathological one? What is the difference between someone who is deemed mentally ill and someone who may consider themselves as having a spiritual experience? Is there a distinct difference between the two? Or is it merely the difference between our cultural understanding and that of others which constitutes these differences? Should we be looking at mental illnesses, particularly psychotic states, in a different light?

These questions continued to follow me even after my time at the Harvard Meditation Research Program. I carried them into my clinical capstone with Professor Daniels, and into a directed study at Susan Whitfield-Gabrieli's EPIC Brain Lab.[5] Under the mentorship of Whitfield-Gabrieli's brilliant grad student, Clare Shaffer, I attempted to develop a conceptual framework to differentiate these "two" complex phenomena—emergent phenomena and psychosis.

In hindsight, my attempt to distinguish pathology from EP became its own kind of koan—a paradoxical question from the Zen tradition meant to expose the inadequacy of rational thought and open the door to enlightenment. I had entered the inquiry question assuming there was a clear boundary between the two, and the deeper I looked, the more those distinctions began to unravel.

What does the DSM have to say?

While the DSM-5-TR (American Psychiatric Association, 2022) does a fine job at conceptualizing different psychopathologies in terms of symptoms and duration, for the most part, the DSM does not consider etiology in terms of diagnosis and instead relies on the concept only in the background. However, the DSM has undergone some revisions over the years to highlight how certain symptoms can arise from mystical practices and be non-pathological in nature. In the section on brief psychotic disorders, the DSM-5-TR states that symptoms should not be included in determining a diagnosis if it is a culturally sanctioned response. In addition, largely thanks to the work of Lindahl et al. (2019, 2020), the DSM-5-TR recognizes that depersonalization/derealization disorder should not be diagnosed if intentionally induced through meditative practices. However, the manual notes that individuals may lose control over these states and develop fear and aversion towards such practices. In Section III of "Emerging Measures and Models," the "Cultural Formulation" subsection considers three different cultural concepts of distress that may influence "symptomatology, help-seeking, clinical presentations, expectations of treatment, illness adaptation, and treatment response." One of these concepts is "cultural explanation or perceived cause," such as the attribution of psychopathology to spirits. The DSM-5-TR acknowledges that all experiences of illness and distress, including those categorized as DSM disorders, are influenced by cultural contexts. As such, the intensity and significance of these distressing experiences should be evaluated in relation to the cultural norms of the individual (American Psychiatric Association, 2022, p. 751).

To aid clinicians in assessing the impact of culture on key aspects of an individual's clinical presentation, the DSM-5-TR provides a set of protocols called the Cultural Formulation Interview. This protocol offers a person-centered approach and considers "Cultural Definition of the Problem; Cultural Perceptions of Cause, Context, and Support; Cultural Factors Affecting Self-Coping and Past Help Seeking; and Cultural Factors Affecting Current Help Seeking." However, much more research is needed to understand emergent phenomena, particularly because their presentation often extends beyond the cultural assumptions embedded in the DSM-5-TR. Findings from Wright et al. (2024, 2025) support the idea that EP can arise across a range of cultural frameworks, even within Western populations. This also highlights the fact that Western societies are not culturally homogenous, making broader subcultural understanding essential.

Thus, as an abiding theme of this chapter, one particular symptomology that DSM renders difficult to discern is the difference between psychosis and certain emergent phenomena such as hallucinations and paranormal beliefs. The DSM-5-TR organizes the schizophrenia spectrum and other psychotic disorders along a gradient of psychopathology, with the primary difference between disorders being the duration during which key symptoms are present. The DSM-5-TR heavily relies on distress and impairment when differentiating between sociocultural normative experiences from symptoms of psychosis, specifically under the categories of "Other or Unspecified Schizophrenia Spectrum and Other Psychotic Disorders" and "Attenuated Psychosis Syndrome," a diagnosis that is currently under consideration (American Psychiatric Association, 2022). This current conceptualization of psychotic disorder within the DSM-5-TR overall alludes to the idea that psychosis is a continuum with varying severity and duration, with strong cultural, spiritual, and religious implications.

Spiritual Emergencies versus Psychopathology—A Transpersonal Perspective

This growing recognition of cultural complexity and diagnostic ambiguity has led some scholars to explore alternative frameworks. One of the first to write about and consider a differentiation between such mystical phenomena and psychopathology was Grof and Grof (1989) in their book *Spiritual Emergency: When Personal Transformation Becomes a Crisis.* Their book offers a rich narrative and provides voices to individuals from various religious and spiritual traditions who have had transcendental experiences. In one of their most recent republished works, Grof and Grof (2017, p. 31) provide a list of criteria that may suggest an individual is experiencing a spiritual emergency. This includes "episodes of unusual experiences that involve change in consciousness and in perceptual, emotional, cognitive, and psychosomatic functioning, in which there is a significant transpersonal emphasis;" "absence of a gross organic brain disorder" and other "physical diseases… which [are] responsible for mental disorder;" "Good general somatic and cardiovascular conditions;" "the ability to see the condition as an inner psychological process;" and "absence of… psychiatric treatment and hospitalization."

Importantly, if the individual is unable to relate to their condition as an inner process, even if the individual meets all other criteria for spiritual emergency, they may not benefit from alternative therapeutic strategies. Grof and Grof (2017, p. 31) also noted that in instances where it is not possible to draw a clear line between a spiritual emergency and psychosis, it might be necessary to experimentally test new approaches—such as transpersonal, humanistic or spiritual therapeutic approaches—before making any final decisions about the strategy of treatment. They also developed a holotropic breathwork technique that combines hyperventilation, sound technology, body work, and music, which they found particularly beneficial in these contexts. While testing for organicity (e.g., a temporal lobe epilepsy) and the way one responds to treatment is certainly a wise place to start in determining a differential diagnosis, it is still very difficult to discern psychopathology from emergent phenomena as there is not one distinct and easily testable biological marker that can reveal a differentiation. In light of this complexity, Grof and Grof (2017) suggest that non-judgmental support combined with a trial-and-error approach using transpersonal or spiritual therapies should be considered before turning to conventional psychiatric interventions.

Grof and Grof's (2017) remarks on the difficulties of making a differential diagnosis are further emphasized in the work of one of their predecessors, Emma Bragdon, a transpersonal psychologist by training whose life work has been dedicated to understanding and educating mental healthcare workers on spiritual emergence and spiritual emergency. In 2013, she founded the Integrative Mental Health University, an online and live educational platform, to help with this initiative.[6]

In one of Bragdon's recorded talks on "How to Differentiate Spiritual Emergency from Pathology"[7] (Bragdon, n.d.), which was largely informed by Grof and Grof's *The Stormy Search for the Self* (1990), she presented a case study of a 28-year-old male from Brazil named Marcelo who was living with his family, had a good social life and no history of trauma. He started to become depressed and was prescribed medication by a psychiatrist; however, his symptoms weren't improving, and he started to hear voices and had a sensation of bugs crawling on his skin. Marcelo was then hospitalized and given antipsychotics, yet he still was not making any improvements. His Catholic parents finally decided to take him to a Spiritist psychiatric hospital.[8]

At this hospital, Marcelo was given a physical examination by a doctor, was assessed by a social worker, and met with a medical intuitive. Organicity and trauma were ruled out as contributing factors to his mental distress, and the mental intuitive could see Marcelo had a great aptitude for energy work and was a channeler of higher information and intelligence. Energy work was voluntarily offered two times a week, where a cleansing of the energetic fields and rebalancing took place, in which Marcelo began training. Throughout this period, Marcelo started to minimize the medications he was taking, ate wholesome foods, exercised, and became affiliated with similar people. Eventually, he was able to live outside the hospital, still on a minimal dose of antipsychotic medication and continuing his energy work training. In a time when the conventional model of care failed Marcelo, this integrative spiritual framework helped him to heal and find greater purpose in life, from which both he and his family benefited. Marcelo's appraisal of his experience was able to shift from negative to positive once he had the right support and framework that allowed him to gain control. Thus, one's initial appraisal of such phenomena is not necessarily a differentiating factor. Just as Wright et al. (2024) contended, the relationship between the valence of one's perceived event and the outcome is not determinative. Another important note is that while Marcelo stabilized, he was still on antipsychotic medication, but this was deemed a spiritual emergence and not pathology, so why would he still need to be on antipsychotics if he was not deemed psychotic? The two often co-exist. It seemed that for Marcelo a combination of Western medicine and esoteric practices was the perfect remedy for his wellbeing.

In her video presentation, Bragdon (n.d.) explained that it is rare for someone to purely go through a spiritual emergence process without any upsets that accompany what we call pathology. One can have a mental illness and a spiritual experience at the same time—that is a part of the human experience. Due to this recognition, in January 2024 Bragdon adapted and updated the differential diagnosis criterion from *The Stormy Search for the Self.* Instead of differential criteria for a "psychiatric disorder" and "spiritual emergence," Emma Bragdon and Tehseen Noorani[9] (Bragdon and Noorani, n.d.) used "criteria indicative of a longer healing process" and "criteria indicative of a shorter healing process." This highlights the fact that while certain aspects may be deemed more "pathological," individuals may still be able to understand their experiences in spiritual terms and integrate this on their road to recovery. Bragdon notes that people's conditions rarely fit into one criterion. However, the more biological, psychological, and social challenges one faces, the longer the healing and integration are likely to be. Bragdon and Noorani broke down the criteria for making this differentiation into three equally important categories: relational, psychological, and biological. An example of relational differentiation between short integration versus long integration is the "[ability] to communicate and co-operate when with a trusted person" and the opposite of that which is "basic mistrust, perception of the world and all people as hostile, persistent thoughts of being persecuted." One of Bragdon and Noorani's (Bragdon, n.d.) six differentiation factors for psychological included "adequate pre-episode functioning as evidenced by interpersonal skills, some success in school and vocation, network of friends, etc," versus "personal history shows long-standing difficulties in interpersonal relationships, such as the inability to make or sustain friendships." Their biological differentiation factors included "negative results of psychological tests for organic impairment of the brain" versus "specific psychological tests indicate organic impairment." As you can see, the latter of each differentiation is indicative of a longer healing process and more "pathological" in nature.

Bragdon's transpersonal approach, growing out of the lifework of Grof and Grof, aims to deconstruct the labels we place on individuals and instead focus on treatment. While this may be an amicable way of viewing such complex phenomena, it is challenging to transfer this approach to general psychology and psychiatry, especially when we rely so heavily on diagnosis to create informed treatment plans and ensure that patients have the appropriate benefits and coverage they need to be functioning members of society. While the rigid boxes the DSM provides may not be so clearly defined, in practice we must learn to work with the labels provided to us, as the DSM's focus on functionality at least aspires toward a type of "objectivity." We may, however, be able to add depth and color to these labels in a way that is expansive. Many mental disorders are already being looked at on a spectrum from "normal" to "pathological," and I believe that this is where our future constructs of mental illness lie. In this way, one may envision a future in which spiritual directors and other mentors can play a more central role in well-being and growth.

Etiology of Psychosis versus Mysticism

In my clinical seminar, I first looked at the tension between psychosis and mysticism from an object relations perspective. The development theories of object relations theorists Donald Winnicott (1896–1971) and Otto Kernberg (1928–) propose that we are all born undifferentiated with only affect tones, but through predictable experiences with caregivers, we build the foundation that then becomes associated with objects, upon which some sense of self eventually emerges. There are many stages that occur throughout development that eventually lead to the stabilization of our ego; however, not everyone achieves these developmental milestones equally, and so some individuals' sense of self is not as fully developed. In other words, we all have a different baseline, and stress and traumatic experiences can cause us to fall down these levels of the psyche-organization, and we can find ourselves in the psychotic state—back to the undifferentiated territory where our development began. This may also be thought of through a Jungian perspective in which the individual attempts to deny the shadows of their ego.

A paper by Crisp (2018) provides an existentialistic perspective in arguing that psychotic experience (PE) exists on a spectrum with "normal" human experience since PE can be experienced by anyone given the right circumstances and context. For instance, one may find oneself having a psychotic-like experience in a spiritual context. Brett (2002) aimed to examine the strikingly similar phenomena of psychosis and mystical experiences with a focus on the delusional mood, a psychological state that is often present in the early stages of schizophrenia. Brett asserts that the delusional mood may be a differentiating factor—albeit an often subtle one—between a longer-term psychotic disorder and more transient and potentially mystical experiences.

Both Crisp (2018) and Brett (2002) agree that an individual with psychosis may have lost their ability to differentiate between self and other, in which they may become socially withdrawn, retreating into the safety of their inner world. However, Brett points out that in Buddhism, this loss of self-from-object distinction isn't viewed as pathological but part of the path of insight into the true nature of reality.[10] Therefore, the inability to distinguish between subject and object may not necessarily be a differential factor between psychosis and mystical experiences. Brett believes that a distinction can be observed in the distorted preservation of the ego structure, along with certain subject/object distinctions. This distorted preservation of the ego structure may also cause an individual's temporality to be distorted, as Crisp (2018) contends that individuals with PE are often preoccupied with the past, anticipate a dreadful future, and fail to anchor their reactions to time and space. From this perspective, psychosis can be viewed as a process of defense—the ego attempting to protect itself from negative emotions. Brett (2002) explains how negative emotional reactions to the distorted preservation can occur when a new ontology (i.e., nature of being) threatens the old ego structure. This may explain why some individuals who experience changes in their sense of self, primarily in the self-other or self-world boundaries, often experience significant distress, which can give rise to emergent phenomena and even psychosis (Lindahl et al., 2017). As Brett (2002) notes, this may arise if the ego structures are not abandoned, and the residual self-identifications and subject/object distinctions are experienced. If attention is turned inward on the subjective experience, the experience will become distorted as the intellect attempts to reestablish objects and reify the self, which may cause one's perception to unify into either the self-constituting-the-world or the world-constituting-the-self.

Crisp (2018) also references another concept that relates to Brett's distorted preservation of the ego: *interpretiveness* and perspective. This concept implies that we are constantly interpreting and re-interpreting previously understood situations across various levels of awareness at a given time. Crisp noted that a combination of stressful or traumatic events and endogenous PE factors may change an individual's capacity to interpret and perceive their experience in a different light. Crisp, quoting Rogers (1959) contends that this is often seen as *a condition of worth* placed by an Other—often an abusive family member—in which the individual's true worth is deeply buried inside, leading to "denied aspects of experiences" that are attributable to "psychotic" behavior. The cure? Crisp suggests "an increase in unconditional self-regard" and a "decrease in the condition of worth," (in Crisp 2018, p. 235) preventing the individual from functioning freely. This may also be related to an individual with PE's tendency to *overcare* when hearing voices, often during periods of stress. However, an individual may begin to realize that the voices are related to their own thoughts and emotions and may represent this Other. This existential perspective may also be looked at from a Jungian lens, in which this Other rests in the shadow that the ego is trying to resist.

Considering the work of both Crisp and Brett, it seems that when ego disillusionment occurs during spiritual or mystical experiences, one must be willing to let go of these ego structures and not attempt to organize these undifferentiated experiences in terms of mundane schema, but to integrate the archetypal shadow in reforming the self. However, there needs to be some structure grounding the individual in their present "illusionary reality." The presence of a well-informed mentoring practitioner or spiritual director with a strong knowledge of cultural contexts would be especially important in reforming the self, particularly if the patient may be having a mystical experience.

A colleague of mine recounted a situation in which a friend of his had become attached to this idea of "no self" or "emptiness." The friend had come to the conviction that everything was an illusion, nothing was real. In an attempt to cure his friend from this illusory reality, he threw a chair at him. His friend ducked his head. If nothing is real, he asked, then why'd you move? This is the sense I make of non-duality. Once one realizes *Heart Sutra's* (c. 3rd–7th centuries CE) assertion that form is emptiness, one must also realize that emptiness is form; form is form; emptiness is emptiness; and everything is just as it is—this is, in the estimation of many Buddhists, the ultimate truth according to Buddha.[11] In other words, it may be that the individual can attain complete ego disillusionment in the altered states of meditation or by other means without attachment and return to the normal mundane reality with these insights still intact. As Brett (2002) contends, this may be thought of as the ability to control attention and maintain emotional balance. The mind may best be viewed as a dynamic system of processes that can function through various modes of existence and, therefore, psychosis may not necessarily result from disease since the alterations in this dynamic system can be intentionally and non-intentionally achieved (Brett, 2002).

Overall, while a spiritual journey through meditation can influence a mystical experience that ruptures the stability of the ego, I found in my research that individuals who had unpleasant and distressing experiences that arose from meditation practice were, in the end, grateful that it occurred. As noted by Stauffer and Capuzzi (2016) in their survey of counseling approaches, existentialists believe that through an existential quest, self-awareness may reveal itself once an individual acknowledges that the world is a subjective construct shaped by their own consciousness. A spiritual awakening may unfold, allowing new hopes to emerge from despair as we peel back another layer in the ongoing revelation of our absolute truth.

In terms of supporting an individual through this spiritual crisis, Crisp (2018) highlighted the importance of the therapist's being-with-others in their journey by focusing on individual personhood and discussing their experiences as normal. Crisp recommended utilizing Prouty's *Pretherapy*, in which reality-based methods are used to help bring "contact-impaired" clients from a pre-expressive state to an expressive state.[12] In this existential approach, the therapist is making contact with the client as one would an undifferentiated baby, holding their hand, helping them find predictable patterns, find meaning, and rebuild the layers of their psyche. This is especially important for individuals who are in a "negative" psychotic state. Or, in the Jungian perspective, through creating a supportive environment, the therapist can gradually facilitate befriending the shadow rather than trying to run and hide from it. For individuals who may be in a more "positive" psychotic state, attached to their spiritual breakthrough and realization of "no-self," this approach may not work. This individual may need further guidance from a Buddhist practitioner or other spiritual director, or maybe just a good friend to snap them back to "reality." Either way, they will require support to help remind them of the non-dualist nature of reality and that while the realization of "no-self" is a great spiritual milestone, the attachment to this state is another illusionary hindrance and cause of suffering.

Differentiating Pathology versus Emergent Phenomena: A Review of the Literature

While a Buddhist perspective and the psychological theories provide useful frameworks and insights into how one may differentiate and support mystical experiences versus pathological ones, they lack rigorous analysis and a general structure or checklist, which many scientists would argue are necessary to validate such claims.

Lindahl et al. (2020) critique Brett's (2002) paper for her lack of empirical research on mystics and the limited number of secondary sources on Buddhist and Hindu traditions, which they argue precluded a close comparison of phenomenology. Lindahl et al. (2020, p. 3) contend that "it is not possible to establish a valid and thorough differentiation of mysticism and psychosis when the phenomenology of psychopathology is based on empirical studies and the phenomenology of mystical experiences is based on religious ideals." This is a huge issue for those researching such phenomena, and scientists are attempting to map these religious ideals and scriptures into their scientific linguistic framework and conceptualization models. Attempting to develop a rigorous model for such loosely defined and highly subjective phenomena reveals a core tension: the unfolding of emergent phenomena resists the rigidity of structural frameworks.

The Lindahl and colleagues paper from 2020 attempted to further differentiate religious and spiritual experiences from pathology through an empirical study using the same data from the Varieties of Contemplative Experiences (VCE) study (Lindahl et al., 2017). They presented a thorough literature review on the topic and formulated their own methods and criteria for differentiating between pathology and spiritual experiences. Utilizing one of the review papers and their own interviews, they developed a combination of theory-driven and data-driven differential diagnostic categories. The categories included: phenomenological qualities, distress, control, duration, impact, functional impairment, health history or condition, critical attitude, circumstances of onset, cultural compatibility, and teachers' skills or resources.

Lindahl et al. (2020) compared the criteria found within ten different studies—including Grof and Grof (2017), Brett (2002), and the DSM-5—for differentiating psychopathologies from religious, spiritual, or mystical experiences. They categorized four of these studies as pertaining to "Spiritual Emergency," and three were categorized as "Mysticism and Psychosis." All studies agreed that phenomenological qualities and duration were possible criteria. Yet Bragdon (n.d.) in her video presentation contended that duration was not a means of differentiating between emergent phenomena and pathology but rather indicative of a longer integrative process. Lindahl et al. (2020) found that the DSM and one other study agreed that distress should be considered as a possible criterion in diagnosis, while three other studies/sub-groups completely rejected this as a possible criterion. Four out of the six studies/subgroups believed control to be a differential factor. In contrast to the studies that highlighted perceived control as a defining distinction, studies on spiritual emergency suggested that even individuals with limited control over their experiences may still be undergoing a transformative spiritual experience rather than a pathological process (Lindahl et al., 2020). Five of the six studies/subgroups mentioned that the impact might need to be taken into consideration in making a differential diagnosis. Lindhal et al. noted that many sources viewed functional impairment as a possible criterion for making a differentiation, but again, some of the studies within the spiritual emergency category rejected this idea. Three of the studies mentioned that health history or condition must be taken into account in making a differential diagnosis, while the rest did not discuss this in their papers. All but the "mysticism and psychosis" subgroup discussed a *critical attitude* as a potential factor in differentiation. Three studies believed the circumstance of onset to be a potential differential factor, while two did not discuss it, and the spiritual emergency category rejected this as a possible criterion. All studies, apart from the mysticism and psychosis subgroup, discussed cultural compatibility as a factor in making a differential diagnosis. What they found through their interviews in their VCE study was a wide range of experiences that received different appraisals depending on the practitioners and teachers and the various Buddhist traditions.

Lindahl et al. (2020) found that while some practitioners argued that appraisal, etiology, level of distress, and impairment are what warrant a differential diagnosis, others disagreed because meditation may trigger a psychotic experience, not a spiritual one. In addition, just because someone has a psychiatric diagnosis this does not necessarily mean that their spiritual experience arising from meditation should be pathologized. Even when phenomena arise spontaneously and are appraised as negative, it does not necessarily mean it is entirely pathological, as we saw in Bragdon's (n.d.) story of Marcelo. However, pathology is often differentiated by levels of distress and for good reason, as this is often indicative that some type of treatment is necessary to stabilize the individual. The issue with this is that Western models of care and spiritual or religious models of care often have different views of what constitutes appropriate treatment for an individual's distress. In a Western context, the instinct is often to suppress these distressing symptoms; however, in certain spiritual and religious contexts, when contained within the structure of a mentored practice, this distress may be viewed as the beginning of a necessary transcendental process. Given these differing frameworks, practitioners investigating or reviewing such experiences should proceed with caution and seek guidance from experienced teachers or mentors to determine the appropriate course of action. A sociocultural informed approach, as well as an ability to recognize distress as part of an inner psychological process, may help in discerning the best path forward. As Grof and Grof (2017) contended, this understanding may serve as a starting point in determining whether intervention should be clinical or spiritual in nature—or quite possibly both. Alternatively, when conventional Western medical approaches aren't working to alleviate the distress, this may be a sign to look towards the spiritual and mystical practices for answers, as seen in the case of Marcelo and many shamanistic journeys described by Grof and Grof (2017).

Overall, mental health professionals must consider multiple factors when conducting a differential diagnosis and deciding on treatment because we are multifaceted creatures. Spiritual directors, meditation mentors, and other religious authorities should also be aware of the subtleties of phenomena displayed by their mentees that these leaders might alternatively fear or dismiss. It is possible that all the factors Lindahl et al. (2020) and the other preliminary work mentioned must be considered when trying to differentiate between a meditative emergent phenomenon and pathology.

Volitional Control of Hallucinations as a Differentiating Factor

As Bragdon (n.d.) aptly stated, "we can't discern psychosis if we haven't decided on what's real and what's unreal"—a reminder that our diagnostic framework is based on culturally sanctioned notions of reality that may not fully encompass the breadth of human experience. Yet during my time at the EPIC Brain Lab, I attempted to find a more scientifically measurable marker to differentiate emergent phenomena from pathology, moving beyond the descriptive criteria I had found in my research. While no instrument can fully grasp the contours of subjective experiences, focusing on one symptom at a time may offer a way to navigate the complexity. As such, I decided that a good starting point would be to explore the differentiation of hallucinations.

I only assessed this question of differentiation in the emergence of hallucinations in meditation and not outside of this context, and therefore, I largely relied on the various research papers by Lindahl and colleagues to guide me. Based on Lindahl et al.'s (2020) paper, there were certain features that Clare and I felt had more weight in making a differential diagnosis, but only for certain phenomenologies. This included duration, control, and critical attitude.

The authors noted that duration could be used as a differential factor for some types of phenomenology, but not all, as the length of experiences varied considerably across different forms of emergent phenomena (Lindahl et al., 2020, p. 10). They defined control broadly as the inability or ability to modulate or stop the experience through behavioral changes such as ceasing meditation or changing one's environment. They noted that certain experiences, particularly somatic ones like Kundalini energy, often persist beyond a meditator's control. In such cases, the degree of control should be considered alongside the specific phenomenology and any behavioral change (Lindahl et al., 2020, pp. 6, 9, 10).

A third criterion, critical attitude, refers to whether an individual maintains intact reality testing and can apply meditative awareness to reflect on and gain insight into their experience (Lindahl et al., 2020, p. 6). The key distinction is in whether they are able to differentiate between consensus reality and internal phenomena (Lindahl et al., 2020, p. 13). A critical attitude was almost exclusively associated with assessing hallucinations, delusions, disorganized thinking, and disruptive behaviors.

Given the wide range of "bizarre" and seemingly "pathological" experiences that may arise from meditation, it is no surprise that different forms of emergent phenomena may require distinct criteria for differential diagnosis.

What counts as pathology versus "normal" spiritual experience is not always consistent and often depends on the specific phenomenology in question.

Even within the broader Buddhist tradition, interpretations of hallucinations differ. In the Theravada tradition, during successful concentration practices, a visual light is expected to arise; however, other visual experiences may be viewed as a red flag for some practitioners. In Zen traditions, hallucinations are not viewed as psychopathology nor warrant an intervention, but an individual must not be seduced by the experience and learn to let it go. Similarly, Tibetan traditions view transient meditation experiences as associated with a range of phenomenology, such as seeing Buddha, and emphasize that one should not get attached to these visions (Lindahl et al., 2020).

This idea of non-attachment is a popular term in Buddhism that "captures an individual's relationship with their experience and highlights a capacity to suspend attempts to control experience through clinging to experiences perceived desirable or avoiding experiences perceived as undesirable whether they are perceived as desirable or undesirable" (Whitehead et al., 2018, p. 1). There is a higher level of consciousness, or awareness, to the experience and the self, in which an individual does not attach themselves to their experience. Based on Buddhist philosophy and Lindahl et al.'s (2020) findings, Clare and I came up with the idea that volitional control, characterized by one's ability to pull oneself out of the experience, may be the difference between pathological hallucinations and meditative hallucinations. We defined control here as a state-level dimension, not a trait, in which awareness, reality testing, and non-attachment may play an influential role in an individual's level of control. In viewing volitional control as a differential factor between pathology and emergent phenomena, we may be able to see how an individual could move up and down like a sliding scale from "pathological" to "emergent phenomena" based on the dimensional state of volitional control they find themselves at in that time.

Neural Networks in the Brain as a Proxy for Volitional Control?

Whitfield-Gabrieli's EPIC Brain Lab has shown how using mindfulness-based training with real-time fMRI neurofeedback reduces auditory hallucinations and modulates resting-state connectivity within the brain's default mode network and central executive network (Bauer et al., 2020). Whitfield-Gabrieli was one of the originators of real-time fMRI (rt-fMRI), a type of biofeedback in which subjects receive feedback information about their current level of activation from a region of interest (ROI) in the brain through a task in which they learn to voluntarily control functional activation of the ROI (DeCharms et al., 2004). Whitfield-Gabrieli's research predominantly focuses on studying the default mode network (DMN), which comprises several functionally connected brain regions and is more active during rest than when performing cognitive tasks. The two main hubs of the DMN, the medial prefrontal cortex (MPFC) and the posterior cingulate cortex (PCC), are believed to mediate self-referential thought, a cognitive process pervasive in everyday life that involves directing attention inward to relate ideas, experiences, and perceptions back to the self. This may include reflecting on one's past or future, or even attempting to synthesize multiple pieces of information into a cohesive narrative.

Another region of the brain, the superior temporal gyrus (STG), has also been shown to play a role in self-referential thinking (Apps and Tsakiris, 2020; Martin et al., 2023; Morfini et al., 2024; Whitfield-Gabrieli and Ford, 2012). The DMN also has been shown to play a role in auditory perception and speech analysis (Binder and Desai, 2011; Li et al., 2018). When performing cognitive tasks, such as reading this tiresome paper, if you are not lost in mind wandering, your DMN should be suppressed. On the other hand, the central executive network (CEN) comprises brain regions that are activated during attention-demanding tasks and is anticorrelated with the DMN (Whitfield-Gabrieli and Ford, 2012). This means when the CEN is "on" the DMN is "off" and vice versa.

A greater magnitude of the DMN-CEN anticorrelation is associated with superior cognitive functions, whereas in schizophrenia, the DMN-CEN anticorrelation is significantly reduced. In addition, the DMN's self-referential nodes, the MPFC and PCC, have been found to be hyperconnected during rest in patients with schizophrenia and major depressive disorder (Bauer et al., 2020; Zhang et al., 2023). These abnormalities within the DMN network have been associated with positive symptoms of schizophrenia (i.e., hallucinations, delusions, disorganized speech, abnormal motor behavior). In schizophrenia patients who experience hallucinations, some scientists have reported increased connectivity between the dorsal MPFC, and the STG compared to non-hallucinating schizophrenia patients (Bauer et al., 2020). Bauer et al. also noted that previous research has shown overactivation of the auditory cortex in the absence of external stimuli for schizophrenia patients experiencing auditory hallucinations. In other words, there is evidence that there is abnormal functioning of neural networks in patients with schizophrenia, and these abnormal neural patterns seem to be specifically related to positive symptoms like hallucinations.

In Bauer et al. (2020), 11 patients diagnosed with schizophrenia or schizoaffective disorder participated in two sessions of fMRI scans. In the first session, patients were trained on mental noting, a component of Vipassana or insight meditation practice. Researchers taught the participants to mentally label whatever experience was most prominent from moment to moment (e.g., hearing, seeing, thinking, feeling). For example, if a participant noticed they were thinking, they would label it "thinking." This helped individuals with the mindfulness meditation by helping them to view their experiences as transient objective events in the mind rather than a true reflection of oneself. The hypothesis of this study was that this type of guided mindfulness would allow participants to also exert some control over their own default mode networks. In turn, participants would experience a reduction in auditory hallucinations. To test this in the second session, patients participated in a real-time neurofeedback task. This task had the individuals look at a screen with two circles, one at the top and one at the bottom, and a ball that they would move by regulating their DMN and CEN through mental noting. The task was to get the ball into the top circle as this was associated with activation of the CEN and deactivation of the DMN. The ball moving downward was associated with higher activation of the DMN and presumably reflecting participants engaging in alternative activities unrelated to mental noting such as introspection or daydreaming.

What is remarkable, and flies in the face of much of how mental health practitioners think of schizophrenia, is that Bauer et al.'s (2020) results showed that there was a significant reduction in auditory hallucination scores one-week post DMN-feedback training. Bauer et al. found a greater reduction in auditory hallucination scores post-neurofeedback, which was correlated with a greater reduction in the STG-MPFC connectivity post-neurofeedback. The results imply that reducing this connectivity within these brain regions by using mindfulness techniques can lead to fewer auditory hallucinations. In addition, all participants successfully reduced DMN activation and increased CEN activation by performing mental noting while receiving real-time feedback.

Patients who learned how to leverage the mindful noting practice to exert better control over their default mode network were able to disengage from their auditory hallucinations and acquired better volitional control over time through mental noting. It may be that the DMN and CEN could act as a neurobiological way of measuring volitional control. However, in regular meditators, we would expect DMN activation to be significantly reduced, yet as I noted regarding emergent phenomena, these auditory and verbal hallucinations can arise because of the practice. This leaves me and others with the question: how do the brains of meditators who experience hallucinations versus the brains of patients with schizophrenia who experience hallucinations differ, if at all? Could it be that the DMN and CEN are anti-correlated in non-pathological hallucinations, while the STG and MPFC are still hyperconnected? What ROIs or neurobiological markers might signify pathology of hallucinations versus this emergent phenomenon? Is the only difference in these experiences between the DMN and CEN, which seems to be a proxy for volitional control? If that is the case, then this mental state of relating to one's experience—that is the subject/object relationship—in an optimal way may be the distinguishing feature between pathology and non-pathological emergent phenomena.

Conclusion

Organicity, as Grof and Grof (2017) contend, may be the first step in discerning general pathology versus emergent phenomena. However, just because someone presents with a physical or neurological abnormality this does not necessarily indicate that it is the primary or only cause of their experiences. A close assessment of changes in one's symptomology is necessary after the physically manifested pathology has been addressed. In the case that one's symptoms don't resolve, further analysis may be needed. A thorough mental status exam could provide useful information and insight into a differential diagnosis.

While the context in which the emergent phenomena arise is important to consider, the difference between one entering a pathological state of psychosis versus non-pathological emergent phenomena may be in the ability to integrate and make meaning of such experience in relation to their ego and their ever-changing self (Crisp, 2018; Lindahl et al., 2020). A cultural, religious, or spiritual framework may provide an individual with a meaningful way of relating to said experience, which may aid them in combating stressful and traumatic experiences and appreciate their interpretiveness and perspective in a new and profound way (Crisp, 2018). While we may not necessarily be able to discern what's real and not real, if the individual is able to ground their experience in a belief system that is comprehensible—however bizarre it may be—and are still able to function in this subject/object relationally driven world, then perhaps their experience is truly non-pathological. Perhaps it is in the maintenance or reshaping of a healthy ego structure along with the integration and re-interpretation of emergent phenomena we are kept sane and grounded in some conceptual if not consensual reality. Since both the ego and DMN are attributed to self-referential thinking, it may very well be that the DMN is the neurobiological marker of the ego—or at least a major part of its function. When the DMN is downregulated, a certain level of ego disillusionment is attained. Perhaps it is in our ever-changing ego structures which either help us maintain volitional control over our experiences or lose it completely.

With the various perspectives I have provided you throughout this essay, you may be able to see how any individual could slide into a pathological state under the right circumstances and ego structures. Of course, more empirical research is needed to support such claims. Nevertheless, I hope that these various perspectives I have provided you throughout this essay have made you ponder this question—what differentiates emergent phenomena from pathological ones?

While the answers aren't clear, one thing is for certain: healing communities—including clinicians, therapists, spiritual directors, meditation leaders, energy healers, and other spiritual practitioners—must learn to come together. Recognizing the non-dualistic nature of existence, they must seek connections between their respective frameworks to better interpret the complex interplay of psychological, physiological, and spiritual phenomena.

A more collaborative approach is necessary. Therapists may need to deepen their sense of spiritual companionship, acknowledging the existential dimensions of healing. Meditation leaders must recognize the importance of containment, ensuring that practitioners are guided safely through transformative experiences. Spiritual directors must remain open-minded, considering that what may initially appear as pathology could, in some cases, be understood through a spiritual lens—alongside the guidance of a psychiatrist.

I have frequently shared these insights with meditation leaders, fellow practitioners, researchers, and laypeople, and their reactions are often a mix of shock, bewilderment, acknowledgement, and moderate skepticism. Yet, almost universally, the response is not dismissal but rather a moment of realization—an "oh wow" moment. Seldom does anyone outright reject the possibility that these perspectives hold truth.

The pursuit of truth is often accompanied by uncertainty, as the distinction between right and wrong is rarely absolute. In a world shaped by perceptual complexities, the search for clarity can lead to moments of disorientation and transformation. Yet, through the process of inquiry—both self-reflective and academic—understanding deepens, and wisdom emerges. This journey is seldom linear; it is a continuous cycle of questioning, revising, and rediscovering. Ideas evolve through reflection and refinement, each revision confronting new uncertainties, peeling back layers of understanding, and revealing that the concept of an absolute truth remains ever elusive, much like the never-ending layers of the psyche.

Notes

1 The concept of the "Other" (uppercase), not "other" (lowercase), can mean many different things. The Other can be thought of as "An Other Person" somewhat akin to Theory of Mind in which we (the observer) understand other people by ascribing mental states to them. However, the Other does not necessarily need to be a person; it could be used to refer to an inanimate object, God, or society itself. Levinas's Absolute Other turns the concept of Other into an encounter with an incomprehensible alterity—otherness. Here the Other is detached from any person or physical entity; yet this Other resonates in every encounter with an other. You will see the term the Other sprinkled throughout this essay, sometimes in reference to "An Other Person" and sometimes as Levinas's abstract Other. The context in which it is applied should give you a clue to which I am referring to. For more information on the concept of the Other, see Benson (2018):

"The other according to Levinas is not just another person but a radical alterity—beyond comprehension or totalization where the other is distinct from self and cannot be reduced to a concept or category. Through encountering the Other we are forced to respond."

2 Christian mysticism may refer to such experiences as the Dark Night of the Soul (see John of the Cross, 1964), a period of deep spiritual desolation that precedes transformation. In Eastern traditions, it may be understood as ego death, the dissolution of mental constructs. Buddhism, frames it as a first glimpse of non-duality—the dissolution of the false separation between truth and illusion, or self and other. From a transpersonal psychology lens, traumatic experiences may break down old psychic structures, paving the way for the emergence of more subtle sensitivities including perceptions of non-ordinary realities, encounters with archetypal figures, and a sense of unity with the cosmos (Grof and Grof, 2017). While terminology varies, the essence remains the same: through suffering, surrender, and

transformation, one emerges with a renewed understanding of existence and a profound connection to something greater than the self.

3 Reiki is considered a unique form of healing energy that practitioners can only channel after receiving a placement or attunement from a Reiki Master. During a session, the practitioner channels the Ki through their hands and performs a byosen scan through the individual's aura. Here the practitioner is looking for hibiki, which can be felt through the palm of the hand as heat, coolness, tingling, pressure pulsating, little electric shocks, discomfort, irregularities, a pulling sensation, or simply an inner knowing. This signifies where there is byoki or unhealthy ki in the body, which is disrupting the energy flow and is believed to diminish the vital functions of organs and cells in our body. Reiki energy is then channeled by the practitioner to these specific areas for healing and another scan is done after treatment to assess its effectiveness by noting the changes in hibiki. However, regardless of where the practitioner places their hands it is believed that the Reiki energy travels through the whole body's fascia which connects the organs and tissues (Rand, 2019).

4 Jhana practices are rooted in Buddhist tradition which focused on developing deep meditative states of concentration that are referred to as *jhanas.* Each *jhana* is characterized by distinct qualities and experiences such as joy, tranquility, and equanimity. For a detailed explanation of jhana states see Gunaratana (1988).

5 The EPIC in EPIC Brain Lab stands for Early Detection, Precision Psychiatry, Innovative Treatments, and Causal Mechanisms. The lab's mission is to understand the brain basis of psychiatric disorders and to translate this knowledge into clinical practice. More information on the research lab can be found at Northeastern University (n.d.).

6 For more information, see IMHU (n.d.a).

7 For the website to the course on how to differentiate spiritual crisis from pathology, see IMHU (n.d.b).

8 Spiritism, developed by Allan Kardec in the second half of the 19th century is deemed a science, philosophy, and religion that explored the nature of spiritual phenomena and believes in reincarnation and karmic principles. Spiritism's popularity resurfaced in Brazil during the 20th century after the "anti-psychiatric hospitalization movement" and Spiritist movement where followers sought to combine conventional medical treatment with complementary spiritual therapies (Lucchetti et al., 2011).

9 Bragdon and Tehseen's table on "*Distinguishing Shorter Spiritual Emergence Integration Processes from Longer Journeys Towards Mental Health*" can be found at IMHU (n.d.b), under the course "*How to Differentiate Spiritual Crisis from Pathology.*"

10 To take the Zen metaphor and progress to insight: Stage 1—Seeing mountain as mountain (self/other separation); Stage 2—Seeing mountain as not mountain (self/other dissolution); Stage 3—Seeing mountain still as mountain (awakening, appreciation).

11 Chapter 2 of the book Dropping Ashes on the Buddha: The Teaching of Zen Master Seung Sahn provides a great explanation and diagram of what this means (Mitchell, 1994).

12 For more information on Prouty's Pre-therapy, see: Psychological Wellbeing (n.d.).

References

Adzic, M., Djordjevic, J., Mitic, M., Brkic, Z., Lukic, I., and Radojcic, M. (2015). The contribution of hypothalamic neuroendocrine, neuroplastic, and neuroinflammatory processes to lipopolysaccharide-induced depressive-like behaviour in female and male rats: Involvement of glucocorticoid receptor and C/EBP-⊠. *Behavioural Brain Research*, 291, 130–139.

Afari, N., Ahumada, S. M., Wright, L. J., Mostoufi, S., Golnari, G., Reis, V., and Cuneo, J. G. (2014). Psychological trauma and functional somatic syndromes: A systematic review and meta-analysis. *Psychosomatic Medicine*, 76 (1), 2–11.

American Psychiatric Association. (2022). *Diagnostic and Statistical Manual of Mental Disorders* (5th ed., text rev). American Psychiatric Association.

Apps, M. A. J., and Tsakiris, M. (2020). The superior temporal gyrus contributes to self and social processing. *Social Cognitive and Affective Neuroscience*, 15(9), 941–950. doi:10.1093/scan/nsaa020

Bauer, C. C. C., Okano, K., Ghosh, S. S., Lee, Y. J., Melero, H., Angeles, C. L., Nestor, P. G., Del Re, E. C., Northoff, G., Niznikiewicz, M. A., and Whitfield-Gabrieli, S. (2020). Real-time fMRI neurofeedback reduces auditory hallucinations and modulates resting state connectivity of involved brain regions: Part 2: Default mode network -preliminary evidence. *Psychiatry Research*, 284, 112770. doi:10.1016/j.psychres.2020.112770

Benson, P. (2018). The concept of the Other from Kant to Lacan. *Philosophy Now*. Available at: https://philosophynow.org/issues/127/The_Concept_of_the_Other_from_Kant_to_Lacan

Binder, J. R., and Desai, R. H. (2011). The neurobiology of semantic memory. *Frontiers in Psychology*, 2, 36. doi:10.3389/fpsyg.2011.00036

Bragdon, E. (n.d.). How to differentiate spiritual crisis from pathology [Online course]. *Integrative Mental Health University*. Available at: https://imhu.org/

Brett, C. (2002). Psychotic and mystical states of being: connections and distinctions. *Philosophy, Psychiatry, and Psychology*, 9(4), 321–341.

Britton, W. B., Lindahl, J. R., Cooper, D. J., Canby, N. K., and Palitsky, R. (2021). Defining and measuring meditation-related adverse effects in mindfulness-based programs. *Clinical Psychological Science*, 9(6), 1185–1204. doi:10.1177/2167702621996340 (Original work published 2021).

Castillo, R. J. (1990). Depersonalization and meditation. *Psychiatry*, 53(2), 158–168. doi:10.1080/00332747.1990.11024497

Cebolla, A., Demarzo, M., Martins, P., Soler, J., and Garcia-Campayo, J. (2017). Unwanted effects: Is there a negative side of meditation? A multicentre survey. *PloS ONE*, 12(9), e0183137. doi:10.1371/journal.pone.0183137

Crisp, R. (2018). An existential ontology for understanding the experience of psychosis. *The Humanistic Psychologist*, 46(3), 230–244. doi:10.1037/hum0000096

DeCharms, R., Christoff, K., Glover, G. H., Pauly, J. M., Whitfield, S., and Gabrieli, J. D. (2004). Learned regulation of spatially localized brain activation using real-time fMRI. *NeuroImage*, 21(1), 436–443. doi:10.1016/j.neuroimage.2003.08.041

Dicks, L. M. T. (2024). Our mental health is determined by an intrinsic interplay between the central nervous system, enteric nerves, and gut microbiota. *International Journal of Molecular Sciences*, 25(1), 38. doi:10.3390/ijms25010038

Dyga, K., and Stupak, R. (2015). Meditation and psychosis. A trigger or a cure? *Archives of Psychiatry and Psychotherapy*, 17(3), 48–58. doi:10.12740/app/58976

Goldberg, S. B., Lam, S. U., Britton, W. B., and Davidson, R. J. (2022). Prevalence of meditation-related adverse effects in a population-based sample in the United States. *Psychotherapy Research, 32(3)*, 291–305. doi:10.1080/10503307.2021.1933646

Grof, C., and Grof, S. (1989). *Spiritual Emergency: When Personal Transformation Becomes a Crisis.* Tarcher.

Grof, C., and Grof, S. (1990). *The Stormy Search for the Self: A Guide to Personal Growth Through Transformational Crisis.* Tarcher.
Grof, C., and Grof, S. (2017). Spiritual emergency: the understanding and treatment of transpersonal crises. *International Journal of Transpersonal Studies.* 36, 30–43. doi:10.24972/ijts. 2017.36.2.30
Gunaratana, H. (1988). The jhānas in Theravāda Buddhist meditation. *Buddhist Publication Society.* Available at: https://www.accesstoinsight.org/lib/authors/gunaratana/wheel351.html.
Hofmann, S. G., Sawyer, A. T., Witt, A. A., and Oh, D. (2010). The effect of mindfulness-based therapy on anxiety and depression: A meta-analytic review. *Journal of Consulting and Clinical Psychology*, 78(2), 169–183. doi:10.1037/a0018555
IMHU. (n.d.a). IMHU: About. *IMHU.* Available at: https://www.imhu.org/manifesto
IMHU. (n.d.b). How to Differentiate Spiritual Crisis from Pathology. *IMHU.* Available at: https://courses.imhu.org/courses/how-to-differentiate-spiritual-crisis-from-pathology
Jacobs, H., and Whitehead, W. E. (2014). A systematic review with meta-analysis of the role of anxiety and depression in irritable bowel syndrome onset. *Psychological Medicine*, 44(12), 2625–2640.
John of the Cross. (1964). *The Complete Works of St. John of the Cross* (K. Kavanaugh and O. Rodriguez, Trans.). Thomas Nelson and Sons.
Kuhn, T. (2012). *The Structure of Scientific Revolutions.* (50th Anniversary ed.). University of Chicago Press. (Original work published 1966.)
Li, J., Wang, J., Liu, J., Meng, X., Zhang, W., and Wang, C. (2018). Effective connectivity within the default mode network in first-episode, drug-naïve schizophrenia patients with auditory verbal hallucinations. *Frontiers in Human Neuroscience*, 12, 529. doi:10.3389/fnhum.2018.00529
Lindahl., J. R., Britton, W. B., Cooper, D., and Kirmayer, L. J. (2019). Challenging and adverse meditation experiences: toward a person-centered approach. In Farias, M., Brazier, D., and Laljee, M., (Eds). *The Oxford Handbook of Meditation.* Oxford University Press. doi: 10.1093/oxfordhb/9780198808640.013.51
Lindahl, J. R., Cooper, D. J., Fisher, N. E., Kirmayer, L. J., and Britton, W. B. (2020). Progress or pathology? differential diagnosis and intervention criteria for meditation-related challenges: Perspectives from Buddhist meditation teachers and Practitioners. *Frontiers in Psychology*, 11, 1905. doi:10.3389/fpsyg.2020.01905
Lindahl, J. R., Fisher, N. E., Cooper, D. J., Rosen, R. K., and Britton, W. B. (2017). The varieties of contemplative experience: A mixed-methods study of meditation-related challenges in western Buddhists. *PLoS ONE*, 12(5). doi:10.1371/journal.pone.0176239
Liu, K., Qin, Z., Qin, Y. (2025) Effects of Reiki therapy on quality of life: a meta-analysis of randomized controlled trials. *Syst. Rev.*, 14, 72. doi:10.1186/s13643-025-02811-5
Lomas, T., Ivtzan, I., and Fu, C. H. (2015). A systematic review of the neurophysiology of mindfulness on EEG oscillations. *Neuroscience and Biobehavioral Reviews*, 57, 401–410. doi:10.1016/j.neubiorev.2015.09.018
Lucchetti, G., Aguiar, P. R., Braghetta, C. C., Vallada, C. P., Moreira-Almeida, A., and Vallada, H. (2011). Spiritist psychiatric hospitals in Brazil: Integration of conventional psychiatric treatment and spiritual complementary therapy. *Culture, Medicine, and Psychiatry*, 36(1), 124–135. doi:10.1007/s11013-011-9239-6

Martin, A. K., Chen, Z., Kohler, M., and French, L. (2023). The medial prefrontal cortex represents self-concept as central to identity. *The Journal of Neuroscience*, 43 (20), 3675–3686. doi:10.1523/JNEUROSCI.0433-23.2023

McManus, D. E. (2017). Reiki is better than placebo and has broad potential as a complementary health therapy. *Journal of Evidence-Based Complementary and Alternative Medicine*, 22(4), 1051–1057. doi:10.1177/2156587217728644

Mikhail, A. (2024). Americans spend an average of $5,300 a year on wellness. From biohacking to walking retreats, here are the top 10 trends driving the market. *Fortune Well*, February 2. Available at: https://fortune.com/well/2024/02/02/americans-spend-5300-wellness-biohacking-2024-tourism-longevity/

Miller, J. J. (1993). The unveiling of traumatic memories and emotions through mindfulness and concentration meditation: Clinical implications and three case reports. *Journal of Transpersonal Psychology*, 25, 169–169. Available at: http://www.brain-health.co/assets/Miller_93.pdf

Mitchell, S. (1994). *Dropping Ashes on the Buddha: The Teaching of Zen Master Seung Sahn*. Grove Press.

Morero, J. A. P., Pereira, S. de S., Esteves, R. B., and Cardoso, L. (2021). Effects of Reiki on mental health care: A systematic review. *Holistic Nursing Practice*, 35(4), 191–198. doi:10.1097/HNP.0000000000000456

Morfini, F., Bauer, C. C. C., Zhang, J., Whitfield-Gabrieli, S., Shinn, A. K., and Niznikiewicz, M. A. (2024). Targeting the superior temporal gyrus with real-time fMRI neurofeedback: A pilot study of the indirect effects on self-referential processes in schizophrenia. *Schizophrenia Research*, 270, 358–365. doi:10.1016/j.schres.2024.06.036

Northeastern University (n.d.). EPIC Brain Lab: Research Mission. Available at: https://whitfield-gabrieli.sites.northeastern.edu/

Peng, R., Wang, W., Liang, L., Han, R., Li, Y., Wang, H., Wang, Y., Li, W., Feng, S., Zhou, J., Huang, Y., Wu, F., and Wu, K. (2025). The brain-gut microbiota network (BGMN) is correlated with symptom severity and neurocognition in patients with schizophrenia. *NeuroImage*, 308. doi:10.1016/j.neuroimage.2025.121052

Popa, L., and Dumitrascu, D. L. (2015). Anxiety and IBS revisited: Ten years later. *Clujul Medical*, 88(3), 253–257. doi:10.15386/cjmed-495

Psychological Wellbeing (n.d.). Prouty's Pre therapy: the essence of contact work – a carer's perspective. *Psychological Wellbeing*. Available at: https://www.psychological-wellbeing.co.uk/?Pre_Therapy

Rand, W. L. (2019). *Reiki: The Healing Touch: First and Second Degree Manual* (Rev. ed.). International Center for Reiki Training.

Reangsing, C., Rittiwong, T., and Schneider, J. K. (2020). Effects of mindfulness meditation interventions on depression in older adults: A meta-analysis. *Aging and Mental Health*, 25(7), 1181–1190. doi:10.1080/13607863.2020.1793901

Rinpoche, Y. M., (2015) What Are the Two Truths [Video]. *YouTube*, April 13. Available at: https://www.youtube.com/watch?v=2ZcCpTwkWsU

Rogers, C. R. (1959). A theory of therapy, personality and interpersonal relationships, as developed in the client-centered framework. In S. Koch (Ed.), *Psychology: A Study of Science: Vol. 3. Formulations of the Person and the Social Context* (pp. 184–256). McGraw-Hill.

Sabe, M., Sentissi, O., and Kaiser, S. (2019). Meditation-based mind-body therapies for negative symptoms of schizophrenia: systematic review of randomized controlled trials and meta-analysis. *Schizophrenia Research*, 212, 15–25.

Schlosser, M., Sparby, T., Vörös, S., Jones, R., and Marchant, N. L. (2019). Unpleasant meditation-related experiences in regular meditators: Prevalence, predictors, and conceptual considerations. *PLoS ONE*, 14(5). e0216643. doi:10.1371/journal.pone.0216643

Schreiner, I., and Malcolm, J. P. (2008). The benefits of mindfulness meditation: Changes in emotional states of depression, anxiety, and stress. *Behaviour Change*, 25 (3), 156–168. doi:10.1375/bech.25.3.156

Shapiro, D. H., Jr (1992). Adverse effects of meditation: a preliminary investigation of long-term meditators. *International Journal of Psychosomatics: Official Publication of the International Psychosomatics Institute*, 39(1–4), 62–67.

Sharma, P., Mahapatra, A., and Gupta, R. (2019). Meditation-induced psychosis: A narrative review and individual patient data analysis. *Irish Journal of Psychological Medicine*, 39(4), 391–397. doi:10.1017/ipm.2019.47\

Stauffer, M. D., and Capuzzi, D. (2016). Human development: Counseling the ever-changing person in context. In *Human Growth and Development Across the Life-span: Applications for Counselors.* (pp. 3–24). John Wiley and Sons, Inc.

Thrane, S., and Cohen, S. M. (2014). Effect of Reiki therapy on pain and anxiety in adults: an in-depth literature review of randomized trials with effect size calculations. *Pain Management Nursing: Official Journal of the American Society of Pain Management Nurses*, 15(4), 897–908. doi:10.1016/j.pmn.2013.07.008

Trivedi, M., Branton, A., Trivedi, D., Mondal, S. and Jana, S. (2024). The use of biofield energy therapy as complementary and alternative medicine in human health care system: a narrative review and potential mechanisms. *Journal of Complementary and Integrative Medicine*, 21(4), 451–460. doi:10.1515/jcim-2024-0027

Wang, X., Shi, X., Lv, J., Zhang, J., Huo, Y., Zuo, G., Lu, G., Liu, C., and She, Y. (2022). Acupuncture and related therapies for the anxiety and depression in irritable bowel syndrome with diarrhea (IBS-D): A network meta-analysis of randomized controlled trials. *Frontiers in Psychiatry*, 13, 1067329. doi:10.3389/fpsyt.2022.1067329

Whitehead, R., Bates, G., Elphinstone, B., Yang, Y., and Murray, G. (2018). Letting go of self: The creation of the nonattachment to self scale. *Frontiers in Psychology*, 9. doi:10.3389/fpsyg.2018.02544

Whitfield-Gabrieli, S., and Ford, J. M. (2012). Default mode network activity and connectivity in psychopathology. *Annual Review of Clinical Psychology*, 8, 49–76. doi:10.1146/annurev-clinpsy-032511-143049

Wright, M. J., Galante, J., Corneille, J. S., Grabovac, A., Ingram, D. M., and Sacchet, M. D. (2024). Altered states of consciousness are prevalent and insufficiently supported clinically: A population survey. *Mindfulness*, 15(5), 1162–1175. doi:10.1007/s12671-024-02356-z

Wright, M. J., Cha, V. L., Streifert, M. R., Ingram, D. M., and Sacchet, M. D. (2025). Risk factors for emergence of sudden unusual mental or somatic experiences and subsequent suffering. *Clinical Psychological Science*, 1–15. doi:10.1177/21677026251330250. Available at: https://meditation.mgh.harvard.edu/files/Wright_25_ClinicalPsychologicalScience.pdf

Zhang, J., Raya, J., Morfini, F., Urban, Z., Pagliaccio, D., Yendiki, A., Auerbach, R. P., Bauer, C. C., and Whitfield-Gabrieli, S. (2023). Reducing default mode network connectivity with mindfulness-based fMRI Neurofeedback: A pilot study among adolescents with affective disorder history. *Molecular Psychiatry*, 28(6), 2540–2548. doi:10.1038/s41380-023-02032-z

Chapter 10

Organizing Desire and Death in Spiritual Direction

A Response to Zecher

Peter Capretto

To occupy space in the humanistic social sciences is to occupy a somewhat principled suspicion toward taxonomies. Like other fields overlapping with the terrain of the social and human sciences, spiritual direction is haunted by the specters of reductionism and the hermeneutic problem of reconciling *Wissenschaft* [knowledge] with human thrownness—specters that the humanistic social sciences must take seriously given the special harm they can wield in clinical settings. Such methodological critiques can tempt us to write off even the most spiritually informed helping professions as fundamentally flawed if they even attempt to organize their thinking through diagnostic or taxonomic structures, as if there were no way to sustain the tension of the double genitive: human science. Such broad methodological critiques have a way of insulating us from the task of reckoning with the lived experiences of others and ourselves, all the while reassuring us that we have taken the higher intellectual road.

Perhaps the most significant assumption built into this suspicion toward taxonomies is the contention that the mere act of organizing experience, desire, and life into a concept or taxonomy is inherently to do violence to it. This is, in an important regard, the central motivation behind the wedding of phenomenological and psychoanalytic methods: whereas our naturalistic attitudes impose unreflective conceptual assumptions onto our experiences of the world and ourselves, practices of resistance analysis and phenomenological bracketing may afford us a less mediated encounter. Not only might this enable us to understand our experience more accurately, but it may prove vital for sustaining an ethical engagement with the other (Levinas, 1969). To embrace this system of taxonomies and diagnostic categories on ourselves would be to move in precisely the opposite direction, the argument goes.

And yet, as historians such as Jonathan Zecher compellingly reveal in this volume and elsewhere (Zecher, 2022), the history of spiritual direction unearths the prospect of taxonomizing desire in such a way that we do not distance ourselves from it, but rather dwell within it in a non-pathological mode that may paradoxically have a freeing effect. For social scientifically inclined humanists, like me, who have long taken joy in deriding anything

DOI: 10.4324/9781003742852-10

that smacks of diagnostic taxonomy, such a prospect for spiritual direction is so counterintuitive that it becomes unclear whether or not it is a doubling down upon the forms of psychological reductionism from which they have been fleeing for decades. Can spiritual direction's tradition of organizing and taxonomizing desire open new possibilities and alliances with humanistic social scientists who see themselves as defending human freedom from the violence of diagnostic reductionism? If so, how does it avoid the well-worn rhetorical pattern of reclaiming premodern philosophical or theological convictions and merely insisting that the historically regressive is in fact the most avant-garde (Milbank, 2006 [1990]; Kotsko, 2009; Raphael, 2006; Rodriguez, 2020; Daniels, 2021)?

What follows is a modest attempt to answer these questions with special attention to Zecher's interdisciplinary contributions in this volume to the history of spiritual direction, particularly in relation to the interaction of emotional life and mortality. Building and borrowing heavily from his insights, I argue not only that spiritual direction's embrace of emotional taxonomies resists the trap of reductionism feared by humanistic social scientists, but also that it would behoove philosophers of language and psychoanalysts to consider spiritual direction a more serious conversation partner on matters of desire, language, and death.

Organizing of Death in Heidegger, Derrida, and Wittgenstein

One of the peculiar emotional experiences Zecher's research in this volume invites me into is the very strange sensation of not finding my characteristic discontent at the idea of emotional taxonomies, but comfort. It is difficult to stress to others how odd of an experience this is for me. I was, and perhaps remain, one of those zealous students of psychology whose primary intellectual identity was: I hate the DSM. And yet here I find myself, maybe for the first time, appreciating the historical prospect of spiritual direction as something that enables us to order emotional life in such a way that does not alienate us from our own experience, but accomplishes precisely the opposite: making ourselves at home in it. I do not yet know what to make of this. It is also not lost on me that one of the characteristic cultural pre-determinations of cishet white dudes is the insistence that others not "put me in a box," because of course I am a special butterfly whom no one understands and yet who transcends all taxonomies. Perhaps as I now age well beyond the midpoint of the lifespan of any man in my family, I find myself listening to Zecher's characterization of Cassian's (1997) emotional taxonomy and thinking to myself with both my identity and mortality in view, "maybe a box would be comfortable."

A curiosity that Zecher's research now elicits from me, then, is the question of what role the quasi-diagnostic quality of spiritual direction's lists plays in its accompaniment of desire in others. Here, I oscillate between sensibilities around the therapeutic function of diagnosis and the identification of emotions. Philosophers of language Martin Heidegger (1889–1976), Jacques Derrida (1930–2004), and Ludwig Wittgenstein (1889–1951)—whose *Lebensform* (or forms of life) Zecher deploys regularly—would both help to flesh out the claim that the linguistic traffic that culminates in particular words invariably shapes not only our understanding of our world, but also our orientation toward our own inner emotional experience of death.

Despite holding rather distinct trainings, social locations, and positions within 20th-century philosophy, Heidegger (2010 [1927]), Derrida (1993), and Wittgenstein (1981 [1922]) make remarkably similar observations regarding the inability for humans to have an experiential encounter with death. Heidegger (2010 [1927], p. 240) notes emphatically, "Dying is not an event" for *Dasein*, nor is it a fact like other facts of one's life.[1] Experiencing the death of others may communicate the biological fact of one's decomposition, which is already in process, but it does not communicate what it means for Dasein to no longer be. In a similar vein Derrida (1993) observes, "Everyone's death, the death of all those who can say 'my death,' is irreplaceable. So is 'my life.' Every other is completely other [*Tout autre est tout autre*]." The irreplaceability of one's death means simultaneously that one cannot die for another and that the fact of another's death tells one nothing about what it means to die one's own. As a result, how to live is in no way informed by the deaths of others. Even if authenticity derives from anticipation of death, others dying around oneself only goes so far to bring this about. The only effect of any death on life will be one's own death on one's own life. If only one could somehow bring such an effect to view.

Death for Wittgenstein (1981 [1922]) is not among the atomistic facts that compose one's world, but nonetheless permeates the world in an unexpected fashion. Similar to both Heidegger and Derrida, Wittgenstein (1981, 6.4211) remarks in the *Tractatus*, "Death is not an event in life. Death is not lived through."[2] Though Wittgenstein is not enticed by the thought of death as an eternal extension of life, that there is life after death, he is open to the possibility that there is life in life, eternally, adding that "[i]f by eternity is understood not endless temporal duration but timelessness, then he lives eternally who lives in the present" (6.4311). The task he insists is that one would live in the present, which strikes one as a new age platitude rather than a statement adhering to his logical world. But considered in light of the present's permeation by the transcendental logic of the world, living in the present might have a more definitive sense for Wittgenstein than a truism. He is insisting that eternity be understood not in the vulgar sense of the term (i.e., endless temporal duration), but rather in terms of a timelessness, a time that abides everywhere and nowhere all at once.

What remains an issue for Heidegger (2010 [1927]), Derrida (1993), and Wittgenstein (1981 [1922]) is the question of the conditions for the possibility for such a relation to the impossible of our own deaths. Beyond merely the recognition of this relation, Heidegger (2010 [1927], p. 246) notes, "We must still ask how the essence of death is defined in terms of the essence of life." This is a question Derrida (1993, p. 28) believes "always remains to be asked." The danger of this question, "How does one experience the relation to the impossible," is its proximity to the question of how one can calculate impossibility. Not only is such an attempt futile, but if one were to succeed, the relation itself would cease with cessation of its incalculability—the impossible is constituted in its incalculability, that it is not limited to the world's calculus. But the other dimension of this question pertains to the simple issue of what it means or how to sustain a relation to the impossible at all.

Time, Derrida (1994, p. 25) stresses in *Specters of Marx*, is "out of joint." This is his response to the question of one's responsibility to the impossible. Experience, one reasons, has boundaries governed by time and space, among many other forms of intuition. And yet, Derrida notes in a primarily descriptive tenor the fact that this is clearly not the case. Like Hamlet's relation to his murdered father, one is haunted by ghosts that are not welcomed, in what Heidegger calls the vulgar understanding of time. Not quite a fact of one's existence, one's responsibility to what one inherits from one's "past" and one's responsibility for what is yet to arrive are for Derrida a given. That is, one is responsible for these alternative events whether one accepts them or not. However, as Derrida stresses through his reference to Heidegger's analysis of death, whether or not one is comported toward these onto-temporal facts of one's existence has a substantial impact on precisely how one will relate to, respond to, and live out the ethical and the political.

Wittgenstein's eternity is not far from Derrida's insistence that our time is out of joint. For time to be out of joint is for the ephemerality of the present to be approached by regions of time that have no place here, presently. Time becomes out of joint in the sense that one becomes implicated in times that one should not be a part of: time before one was born and time that has not yet been. But to be implicated or born to an inheritance does not mean that one "bear[s] any less of a responsibility" (Derrida, 1994, p. 24). Regarding the past, one bears responsibility for what precedes oneself. To say that one inherits is not simply to say that one is born to a context which one cannot but take on—a thrownness—but that one is called on "to render justice, and to redress history" (Derrida, 1994, p. 24). One is responsible for "the *wrong* of history" (Derrida, 1994, p. 24). Derrida is pointing to the fact that the inheritance of time demands an insatiable responsibility. Inheritance itself poses an ethical challenge. It is as if one's own birth is itself an interpellation of history in its movement of violence and injustice. One's birth is thrown at and into history, as if to interrupt, but instead to be given an inheritance by history itself: "You have interrupted me with your birth? Here is my response and my gift to you, one which will haunt you into the unforeseeable future, an inheritance" (Derrida, 1994, pp. 24–25). One's inheritance is itself an arresting of time, and the arresting of oneself in time.

For Wittgenstein, the limits of language only do so much to insulate experience from what exceeds it. Like Heidegger, Wittgenstein (1981 [1922], 6.522) recognizes that "There is indeed the inexpressible. This *shows* itself; it is the mystical." Wittgenstein's mystical, which Derrida references, is the view that the inexpressible shows itself in and through experience. This position on its own does not seem to address the question of how this occurs any better than Heidegger, who leaves the question unresolved. The logic of Wittgenstein's world seems to preclude anything like an excess or an overflow of facts. The unanalyzable is merely the unsayable, and one ought not try to explain it. However, logic is not something that one experiences like a fact. He notes enigmatically, "Logic is not a theory by a reflexion of the world. Logic is transcendental" (Wittgenstein, 1981 [1922], 6.13). It is this type of remark that troubled Wittgenstein's contemporary logical positivists so much. There appears to be no room in philosophy to discuss the transcendental, especially considering how tightly knit Wittgenstein's propositions describe the analyzable world. Yet Wittgenstein understands that one does not have a clear understanding of the founding of logic in the world. The mystical foundation of logic is that one has no sense of precisely how logic has come to have such a profoundly governing force on one's world. One finds oneself incessantly in relation to logic, but this is a thrown relation. "Logic *precedes* every experience—that something is *so*. It is before the How, not before the What" (Wittgenstein, 1981 [1922], 5.552). One cannot describe a time before logic's reign. One is thrown into it. For Wittgenstein, the What of logic is the manifest content of one's world. To remark that "[t]he world is the totality of facts, not of things," indicates for Wittgenstein that there is indeed a profound whatness to the logic of the world (Wittgenstein, 1981, 1.1). One is, in fact, caught in a place where it seems improper to ask the question of "How" logic has its effect on the world. To do so would require a departure from the Heideggerian "this-worldly" character of such an analysis, with which Wittgenstein seems to agree.

But in the company of the mystical, Wittgenstein betrays such a simple reading of his respect for the anteriority of language to the How. Logic does precede the how of the question, but he remarks, "[L]ogical propositions describe the scaffolding of the world, or rather they present it" (Wittgenstein, 1981 [1922], 6.124). Logic is at once transcendental, in the form of logical propositions, and descriptive of the world's *Gerüst*, scaffolding or matrix. For a proposition to be meaningful and to have sense, it must adhere to this logical scaffolding. Not completely dissimilar to a color, which in its abstracted form cannot become manifest in a world—there is no such thing as "red" but only red *things*—logic is something of which one cannot have a pure sense, yet one finds everything meaningful to be permeated thereby.

Wittgenstein of course would not concede that all questions, simply by virtue of being able to posit them, are sensical and derivative of analyzable facts. In the *Tractatus*, he famously concludes, "Whereof one cannot speak, thereof one must be silent" (Wittgenstein, 1981 [1922], 7). But the ways in which he runs up against this limit of speech become increasingly apparent and divergent in his middle and later years. He revises his thesis when he writes to himself, "Don't *for heaven's sake*, be afraid of talking nonsense! Only don't fail to pay attention to your nonsense" (Wittgenstein, 1998, p. 64). As for Derrida and Heidegger, one can only respect the limits of experience to a certain point, notably when experience shows the effects of something not originating in experience. The task of paying attention to one's nonsense is then the task of holding a critical lens to what one believes effects one's life nonsensically. It would require more than simply gesturing to the fact that one's death is nonsensical, but actually laboring to explain how the nonsensical makes its way into life's edge.

This imperative, to mind one's nonsense, then brings one full circle to the unresolved question in Heidegger and Derrida regarding how the effects of death are defined in terms of life. Wittgenstein's image of the scaffolding or matrix of the transcendental is a helpful way to articulate that the transcendental is related to the imminent as a structuring of sorts. Like a law with mystical foundations, death and ethics are already at work in one's life, structuring not only the absolute features of one's life such as one's decomposition, but even the rudimentary details such as how long one is expected to work before retiring. "The inexpressible (what I find enigmatic & cannot express) perhaps provides the background, against which whatever I was able to express acquires meaning" (Wittgenstein, 1998, p. 23). Becoming attuned to these details is the start of what it would mean to live authentically and resolutely toward not only one's death, but the infinite demands of an ethical and political inheritance that would seem as foreign as death itself. To take this explanation any further than this open attunement to the effects of the transcendental ethic would require an anteriority to the founding of its imminence for one's this-worldly analysis. Wittgenstein (2001 [1953], p. 43) thus writes in the *Philosophical Investigations*:

> Philosophy simply puts everything before us, and neither explains nor deduces anything.—Since everything lies open to view there is nothing to explain. For what is hidden, for example, is of no interest to us. One might also give the name 'philosophy' to what is possible *before* [*vor*] all new discoveries and inventions.

Wittgenstein would perhaps contend, then, that there is no explaining the how of the relation of the impossible or the nonsensical to the world. Ethics's transcendence means that one's this-worldly analysis will forever, timelessly, remain unable to explain precisely the effect that it has on one presently.

How the essence of death is defined in terms of life is for Derrida bound up with the question of how the future is germane for experience in the present. But for Wittgenstein as much as for Heidegger, this How remains more than "to be asked," but to be explained. Wittgenstein's sense of the transcendental scaffolding of ethics and logic is a helpful lens for working with being toward the impossible. Heideggerian authenticity in this scheme would require an attunement to this scaffolding, to the way in which the impossible permeates the world with a matrix that provides a mystical governance of possibility. As one might expect, the impossible in this approach refuses the desire to understand its How, but instead calls for closer attention to its effects, which are nothing less than the radical and mystical structuring of one's world.

Taxonomizing Desire in Spiritual Direction

Yet within the specific context of spiritual direction, Zecher's engagement with the emotional taxonomies of Cassien in this current volume also raises a challenging series of questions in response to the transcendental scaffolding offered by Heidegger, Derrida, and Wittgenstein. That is, if Zecher is correct that the fundamental task of spiritual direction is to assist someone with their own developing relationship with the divine, what does it imply about that aim that the primary method for accomplishing this is the translation of otherwise formless affective energy into more regulated and diagnostic emotional categories? Similarly, if the pastoral theologian Pamela Cooper-White, also in this volume, is correct in her reading of the poet Mary Oliver (1990, p. 60) that a guiding question for spiritual direction is the pursuit of the question, "what is it you plan to do/ with your one wild and precious life?", then what consequence do directors have upon directees if and when they invite them to the revaluation of their relation to the divine through such emotional taxonomies? More to the point, if the method of spiritual direction is correct in utilizing emotional taxonomies to discern what to do with one's precious life, what does this imply about God's desire for our desire?

In this volume, Zecher notes the ways that Cassian (1997 [c. 430]) built upon Evagrius's work of listing eight principal "thoughts" that in more contemporary parlance quite clearly register as emotions such as sadness, anger, and acedia. More than a mere effort to systematize, the benefits of such a taxonomy include the ability to reveal both the interrelation of these emotions and their contours in relation to one another. "The lists enable spiritual direction by giving director and disciple a common language and reference," Zecher, in this volume, helpfully explains. Insofar as spiritual direction remains committed to cultivating a relation to the divine, taxonomizing emotion and desire may very well be providing that transcendental scaffolding alluded to by Wittgenstein, Heidegger, and Derrida—1500 years before they would.

The root of the discourse over whether or not to taxonomize desire goes to the heart of the original controversy of the idea of a human science and that specter of reductionism, which here one encounters with the reductionism of language itself in its capacity to give voice to human emotion and perhaps even a transcendental scaffolding to encounter death in any substantive fashion. The idea of a human science is unsettling to many not because it is a contradiction of terms, but rather because it has the courage to inquire into what remains most enigmatic in human inquiry itself. That is, to pursue something like a human science is to accept Freud's (1966 [1917], p. 31) invitation to sustain attention on "the inconsiderable events which have been put aside by the other sciences as being too unimportant." This means dwelling with the parts of ourselves—the drives, traumas, attachments, and prospective losses—that cannot be operationalized by behaviorism or cognitive science. The audacity of a human science is thus its willingness to claim this "unimportant" remainder as the greatest horizon for insight, understanding, and care. This is why a discipline like psychology practiced as human science is, in fact, less abstract and more practical than cognitive behaviorism: it rejects theory that distances the clinician from the emotional world of those for whom they claim to care, and invites an even more demanding ethical call.

This conundrum may be felt in its greatest force in the question of whether finding language clarifies or kills desire. Each of us has likely had the experience of learning a new word, concept, or emotion that captures an experience or mental state for which we previously had no vocabulary. The arguably therapeutic function of language then becomes the process of taking otherwise chaotic psychic energy and finding a home for it within the structural language games that order one's life. Consider a plausible experience in the discovery of new emotional language for yourself. You have lived your whole life in a heightened state of emotional dysregulation during certain times of the day, only to learn a word called being "hangry," which suddenly clarifies the genesis of several arguments you've had with peers and loved ones in the late afternoon in recent years. Something that previously felt intense and overwhelming no longer feels this way, and like we might now be at home with it. Vocabulary itself then compels you to repentance, and to carry a Snickers in your briefcase.

However, the question for me remains: by taxonomizing one's experience in this way through language, has one become more attuned to one's desire? Or, is the relief felt by finding the language for an experience more accurately understood as the satiation of desire through its erasure? Working heavily from Lacan's (2006 [1996], p. 737) famous position that "the unconscious, which tells the truth about truth, is structured like a language," philosopher Richard Boothby (1991, p. 227) notes that there is a "knotting of desire, death, and language" that must be reckoned with in this question. More specifically in his interrogation of Lacan's retrieval of Freud, Boothby (1991, p. 131) argues, "What makes this project especially challenging is that its objective is not merely to show the compatibility of desire and language, but also to show how they are necessarily and inextricably bound up with one another." This process of translating emotional life to language, as I have just laid it out, appears quite plainly to be a process of putting desire to death. Those moments of relief one found when one learned that special word that captured an inchoate emotional experience that had been building without full awareness are, now that one thinks upon them, moments of the attenuation of desire. If the philosopher Guy Thompson (2017, p. 91) is correct that "psychopathology may simply mean an occasion of spiritual suffering, mental anguish, soul murder, or the death of desire," then it remains unclear if taxonomizing emotion helps or exacerbates our conditions. Language, lists, and diagnoses may all function this way as the death of desire.

Yet Boothby (1991, p. 110) complicates matters further in noting that "the function of language appears in the role of a liberating influence, which opens up the possibility of testing a foreclosed and forbidden jouissance." That is, language may function as a certain death of desire, but it also creates space for us to inhabit an encounter with desire that risks our own undoing. This makes sense for people like Hegel and Lacan: of course desire seeks to kill itself; desire makes us self-conscious and uncontained; the ego always seeks organization and self-certainty as a way of mitigating its own vulnerability and annihilation. Hunger always pursues its own erasure. Perhaps spiritual direction may find itself better allied with psychoanalysis, phenomenology, and the philosophy of language than immediately hits the eye.

I am tempted to suggest that the old, DSM-hating version of myself was right: diagnosis always deprives us of our capacity to emotionally dwell with ourselves in the world. However, Zecher's work now invites me to consider whether spiritual direction is onto something, namely: taxonomizing emotions is part of a necessary process of kenosis, whereby we empty ourselves of desire, attenuate self-consciousness, and align our inner worlds to the divine.

Notes

1 This and all subsequent citations to Heidegger's *Being and Time* refer to the original German pagination.
2 This and all subsequent citations to Wittgenstein's *Tractatus* refer to the standardized outlining system he originally employed.

References

Boothby, R. (1991). *Death and desire: Psychoanalytic theory in Lacan's return to Freud*. Routledge.

Cassian, J. (1997). *The conferences* (B. Ramsey, Trans.). Ancient Christian Writers 57. Newman Press. (Original text completed c. 430.)

Daniels, A. B. (ed.) (2021). *Dante & the Other: A phenomenology of Love*. Psychology & the Other Series, Routledge.

Derrida, J. (1993). *Aporias* (T. Dutoit, Trans.). Stanford University Press.

Derrida, J. (1994). *Specters of Marx: The state of debt, the work of mourning and the new international* (P. Kamuf, Trans.). Routledge. (Original work published 1993.)

Freud, S. (1966). *Introductory lectures on psycho-analysis*. (J. Strachey, Ed. and Trans.). W. W. Norton and Company. (Original work published 1917.)

Heidegger, M. (2010). *Being and time* (J. Stambaugh, Trans.). SUNY Press. (Original work published 1927.)

Kotsko, A. (2009). "That they might have ontology": Radical orthodoxy and the new debate. *Political Theology*, 10(1), 115–124.

Lacan, J. (2006). Science and truth (B. Fink, Trans.). In *Écrits.* W. W. Norton and Company. (Original work published 1966)

Levinas, E. (1969). *Totality and infinity: An essay on exteriority* (A. Lingis, Trans.) Duquesne University Press. (Original work published 1961.)

Milbank, J. (2006). *Theology and social theory: Beyond secular reason.* (2nd ed.). Blackwell. (Original work published 1990.)

Oliver, M. (1990). *House of light.* Beacon Press.

Raphael, M. R. (2006). Standing at a demythologised Sinai? Reading Jewish feminist theology through the critical lens of radical orthodoxy. In R. Radford Ruether and M. Grau (Eds.), *Interpreting the Postmodern: Responses to 'Radical Orthodoxy'* (pp. 197–214). Continuum.

Rodriguez, R. R. (2020, July 16). A "themed identity" theologian responds to John Milbank. *Political Theology Network.* Available at: https://politicaltheology.com/a-themed-identity-theologian-responds-to-john-milbank/

Thompson, G. (2017). *The death of desire: An existential study in sanity and madness* (2nd ed.). Routledge. (Original work published 1985.)

Wittgenstein, L. (1981). *Tractatus logico-philosophicus* (C. K. Ogden, Trans.). Routledge. (Original work published 1922.)

Wittgenstein, L. (1998). *Culture and value* (2nd ed.) (G. H. von Wright, Ed.; P. Winch, Trans.). Blackwell. (Original work published 1977.)

Wittgenstein, L. (2001). *Philosophical investigations* (3rd ed.). (G. E. M. Anscombe, Trans.). Blackwell, 2001. (Original work published 1953.)

Zecher, J. L. (2022). *Spiritual direction as a medical art in early Christian monasticism.* Oxford University Press.

Chapter 11

A Response to Zecher

Aaron B. Daniels

Jonathan Zecher's examination of the context and roots of John Cassian's (c. 360–c. 435) description of the Desert Fathers is deep and thick with implications. Zecher skillfully offers his readers ample descriptions of the preceding philosophical, spiritual, and medical currents informing what commentators typically cast as the first practice of spiritual direction in the Christian tradition. Zecher invites his readers to reconsider what such essential concepts as emotion, rationality, and transformation meant 16 centuries ago. For this response, I invite readers to extend this reconsideration to what these sorts of terms may mean today, starting—and eventually ending—with "spiritual direction."

"Spiritual direction" has accumulated many definitions, and this current volume speaks to a healthy range of them. This diversity of characterizations likely signals an even broader range of actual practices. Moreover, that breadth is expanding exponentially in concert with growing interest in this art. Although the practice is indisputably ancient, an examination of scholarly databases reveals a telling trend. Searching 40 databases of scholarly sources covering humanities, religion, philosophy, medicine, media, and the social sciences, of the almost 4,000 articles with "spiritual direction" as a search term, reaching back to 1882, more than half have been published in just the last 20 years. To add complexity to the investigation of this range of practices, the term "direction" isn't universally adopted, as words like "accompaniment," "companionship," "guidance," or even "coaching" vie with the more widely used and long-standing "direction." And as applications of mindfulness, wellness, and more humanistic and/or non-Christian approaches grow, even the word "spiritual" in all its ambiguity can cease to adequately convey the practice.

Perhaps it is best that scholars do not seek to establish one universal definition, but to develop a discourse by which we can discuss the nuances. Building on this legacy, this current volume of essays is another effort to offer more collected perspectives to this scholarship and to further expand the breadth and depth of voices.

As scholars and practitioners debate terminology, one of the most abiding and beloved definitions for the practice of spiritual direction is the Irish

DOI: 10.4324/9781003742852-11

Gaelic term *anamchara*, often written *anam cara*—that is, "the soul's friend." Though a long-standing concept within Celtic Christianity, the term came to greater popularity with John O'Donohue's (1956–2008) work, *Anam Cara: A Book of Celtic Wisdom* (O'Donohue, 1997). O'Donohue offers a rich, deep, warm, and Creation-affirming vision that appeals to many in the profession. Yet, if the "spiritual" in spiritual direction gives many pause in terms of definition, then what can we do with the "soul" in "soul's friend"?

One popular conception, certainly in the post-Spiritualism era in which we live, is to cast the soul as some sort of glowing, eternal version of ourselves. Here, "Spiritualism" is not the same thing as the far broader term "spirituality." My use of "Spiritualism" here refers to the cultural phenomena of séances, mediums, hauntings, and a host of questionably appropriated religious concepts of reincarnation, after-life cosmologies, and world (pre)histories emerging in the mid-1800s. Undeniably drawing on various mystics, such as Emanuel Swedenborg (1688–1772), it is, however, the folk-movement catalyzed with the Fox Sisters in 1848 that leads to widespread belief in very specific types of afterlives and the ability to contact spirits. It is this Spiritualism which will feed into and spur various magical and occult revivals, cobbled together Western esotericisms, and eventually the New Age spirituality of the 20th century. Moreover, the larger cultural effects of Spiritualism have far outlasted and reached far beyond the bounds of table-tapping and Ouija boards.

Arguably, it is Spiritualism's sort of nearly ectoplasmic soul that has been patched onto various religions' cosmologies and theologies as that which might go to heaven, hell, purgatory, or some form of afterlife. Perhaps it is unfair to heap all the blame on the Spiritists or Spiritualists for this vaguely see-through version of ourselves. After all, doesn't Dante (1265–1321) offer copious spiritual consequences for something very much like these souls in his *Commedia*? But regardless of the origin and development of this construct of the soul, we might do well to question the effect of this conceptualization of soul on what a soul's friend might be and what the work of soul is.

I refer to Dante specifically because, as I and other authors emphasize elsewhere (Daniels, 2021), Dante exists just on the cusp of the European Renaissance. This places him as pre-modern, if only just. This soul with which we most popularly wrestle today is decidedly modern in its conceptualization. The modern soul onto which the Spiritualists heaped their conceptualizations is the strange remainder left over from Descartes's (1596–1650)—and others'—enshrining of the mind/body split equation. For Dante, three centuries before Descartes, this is not quite the psychotheocosmology through which he guides his readers. Take, for example, Canto XIII of *Inferno*, which heartbreakingly portrays the fate of those who have taken their own lives.

Dante and Virgil reach a thick wood filled with thornbushes. Under Virgil's mentorship, Dante discovers that these thornbushes are actually the souls of those who have committed suicide. When Dante breaks off a twig, the sap that bubbles forth is their blood—blood that speaks in the agony of the damned. Promising that their story will live on if they tell their tale, Dante learns that, at the Christian Rapture,

> Like other souls, we shall seek out the flesh
> that we have left, but none of us shall wear it;
> it is not right for any man to have
> what he himself has cast aside. We'll drag
> our bodies here; they'll hang in this sad wood,
> each on the stump of its vindictive shade.
> (Alighieri, 1320, *Inferno* XIII:103–108,
> Mandelbaum Translation)

And later, another soul explains "I made—of my own house—my gallows place" (Alighieri, 1320, XIII:151). Dante is bridging two visions of the End of Days. On one side is a Resurrection of the Flesh in which the deceased sleep until the Second Coming when they may be raised from the dead. The other image is of souls that live on without a body in a provisional afterlife until the Final Trumpet Call ends the world and makes permanent one's spiritual residency. For Dante's hybrid vision, in Canto XIII, the shades of the dead who have taken their own life are to be united with their flesh; but it will not take on new life. It will hang on the thornbush of their "vindictive shade."

Teodolinda Barolini (2018) in her *Commento* on Canto XIII emphasizes "the inseparable personhood of soul that is embodied and of body that is ensouled" and "the indestructible unity of body and soul." That is to say, in spite of my quip about Dante introducing incorporeal souls, it is alien to Dante's cosmology to speak of body and soul as ultimately separate. Moreover, the separation may be pathological—a signification of an untenable state that seeks resolution by whatever means possible.

Dante's Canto XIII in *Inferno* is rife with wordplay pointing to essential insights. It begins with a series of grammatical negations to describe the landscape—negations that foreshadow the bitter denials intrinsic to Dante's conceptualization of suicide. Later, Dante creates an Italian tongue-twister repeating various forms of the verb *credere* [to believe]—letting the reader know that belief and clutching to cherished convictions are at play. And the dense thorny landscape itself echoes the *selva oscura* [dark woods] in which Dante initially came to himself in Canto I:1 of *Inferno*. I briefly mention these aspects to underline that Dante is a poet first and a theologian in service of poetry. Yet, as a poet, he may be imminently more qualified to address matters of soul—of soulfulness—than many theologians.

With these matters in mind, our attention turns now to Zecher's marvelous guided tour of the landscape of the Desert Fathers and Mothers through which John Cassian himself takes his readers—and, in doing so, links us still further back into the Stoics and ancient Greek medicine. To give some historical context to Cassian's writings which he undertook around 420CE, this is the early Christian church. The Apostle's Creed emerges between 120–250CE and a Creed of Nicaea is set in 325CE, but the Nicene Creed will only come about in 381CE. Nonetheless, the infamous *filioque* [Latin: and "from the Son"] that would accelerate the separation of Eastern and Western Christianity was not yet in play. Constantine had only issued the Edict of Milan, ending Roman persecution of Christianity, in 313CE; and the Edict of Thessalonica making Christianity the Roman Empire's state church comes only in 380CE. All this is by way of saying that Christianity is much more a collection of movements than it is any sort of institution. "Doctrines" and "heresies" dance and change places while regional variations abound. Therefore, Cassian's writings exist in a dynamic landscape. He writes to try to clarify, build, and guide. In this doctrinal churn, there is already something of a pining for an assumed clarity and simplicity that came before—notably since Cassian is not listed among the Desert Fathers yet seeks to let them inform Christian practice and guidance.

To provide current context: within Christianity, the Desert Fathers and Mothers are credited with the origin of the practice of spiritual direction. This statement is repeated so often in literature and trainings as to be an article of faith. With this origin story in place, spiritual direction is a unique, guiding relationship focused on the development of the individual. Historically, confession may have played a critical role, but with lay directors making up a large portion of practitioners, the Desert Fathers and Mothers can be taken up as examples of something other than solely confessor, priestly guide, or faithful friend in conversation. That this origin story forecloses a larger context extending beyond Christianity does not receive mention in any account of the practice I have read.

Thus, how important it is that Zecher tells us that this discourse stretches back into pre-Christian sources. Can the reader of today read passages about "vices," "passions," or parts of the "soul" with anything like fresh eyes? This is, in part, what Zecher asks of us. Today, we undoubtedly face a mental health crisis. Whether it is new, newly labeled, exacerbated, or a recasting of a long-term crisis are questions for other essays and other authors to discern. But what Zecher offers us is nothing less than a call to think in very new (i.e., very old) ways about healing, medicine, diagnosis, and therapy—and, if I may add, soulfulness. In doing so, might we at least come to think differently about our "mental health" and whatever this current crisis is?

Perhaps, like me, until reading Zecher's chapter, the most you've read of the Desert Fathers and Mothers is Thomas Merton's slim volume *The Wisdom of the Desert: Sayings of the Desert Fathers of the Fourth Century* (Merton, 1960). Merton's selections, translations, and arrangement of his content take on a decidedly Zen tone. Merton sets out these passages as *koans*—meant to short circuit the busy mind's efforts to label, explain, and contain experience. Zecher's writings are a decided and long-needed alternative reading. And, since Zecher provides us with ample context, connections, and legacies, rather than Merton's stark sampling, one could certainly see Zecher's reading as far better justified. Furthermore, as I hope this response can insinuate, Zecher's interpretation is more soulful than Merton's.

An implication threads throughout Zecher's encyclopedic treatment of Cassian's thought—and that is of how a fundamental impulse may take many shapes based on how we take it up and direct it. I have to be careful, however, not to over-extend this sentiment. I do not read Zecher to be asserting that only a short step will take the reader to Aquinas or Dante in which the same fundamental impulse can be disastrously twisted into vice, or wrestled with in the work of spiritual purgation, or ultimately liberated into its truth in virtue. Readers of Dante's *Commedia* know that down into hell, through the center of the earth to the other side, up the Mountain of Purgatory, and into the Celestial Spheres, Dante essentially describes a straight vector. It may coil in Hell and Purgatory, but the entrapping, desperate lust of Hell, gives way to the burning Purgatory fire, which yields the journey into the sublime Love of Paradise. And to state it again, that is not the Desert Fathers' and Mothers' vision a full millennium before Dante. Thus, I do not read Zecher asserting that the same impulse drives virtue and vice for Cassian and his subjects.

But perhaps it is accurate to say that affects are fundamental to our souls. These passions don't simply translate from body to soul or spirit—or from spirit and soul to body. Rather, this is a unified field which demands something quite different than a top-down emphasis on asserting cognitive control. Nor does one simply, bottom-up, balance one's humours with a proper diet and physical discipline to realign the passions. Here is a re-membering of our dismembered psyche—that is our soul.

This is a landscape where trains of thought(s) emerge from trait-like configurations of the organs of psyche (i.e., the soul's passions). And these organs are embodied—so much so that the term "embodied" implies an extra step than this psychotheocosmology merits. Perhaps more shocking by more 20th century humanistic standards is Zecher's observation (in this volume) that spiritual direction—in Cassian's continuation of the Desert Fathers' and Greek Medicine's model—involves "a transplant operation, with the director working surgically on emotional dispositions and the values that underpin them." I was tempted at first to borrow Hillman's acorn theory from his *Soul's Code* (Hillman, 1996) to think of Cassian's model. However, these Desert Fathers are not seeking to cultivate one's *daimon* to develop in the most salubrious of fashions. Instead, they must indeed get to such a deep level of the impulses, ferreting out lines of felt-reasoning, to reveal what misleads one—not merely to redirect, but to welcome a reconfiguration, a rebirth. And only from there can the re-membering and rearrangements occur. This is a depth undertaking to be sure, but one in which the soul must be first laid open.

So, if the contemporary reader grants that only a narrow band of today's spiritual directors are audacious enough to take such a radically directive transplant approach, what might we do with this discourse Zecher describes so well? If we take something like a reconstructionist approach—borrowing from Rabbi Mordecai Kaplan—and let the past have a vote but not a veto, we can find a way to take up this discourse that can shock us into new ways of thinking of this work of spiritual direction and how to be a friend to soulfulness.

Spiritual direction runs the risk of supporting the overly convenient partitions in our lives—the dismembering to which I refer above. I go to my therapist to address my psychopathologies. I go to my pastoral counselor to work through emergent crises in my life utilizing faith-based tools. I go to my physician or a physical therapist to deal with my bad back. I see a vocational counselor to think through my career. And so on. Most spiritual directors I've met weave a careful dance as they try to challenge these often-rigid divisions while also avoiding practicing well beyond their competency. Typically, the directee takes the lead and the director then opens up the discourse into which the directee invites them. (Here we can see the clearest case for why the director/directee language is rather more fluid than some might think.)

One phrase that I have received from my director and used with my directees speaks to an essential shift with regard to this compartmentalization: "How do you invite God into this part of your life?" The phrasing can shift to "welcoming," or "acknowledging," or "expressing gratitude to" God within some aspect of our lived world. For more deistic directees, it leans to acknowledging; for more mystical work, it may be about opening a part of our lives to the Ineffable. I think that my Wiccan—and many Christian—friends certainly see the value in welcoming the Mother's love into a part of our lives in which we have hitherto not acknowledged this Presence.

What impresses and touches me about this turn of phrase—and turn of soul—is that it reaches beyond. Of course, like the devoted Imaginal Psychologist I am, I want my directees to deepen their soulfulness—to dwell in the messiness of their lives, their conflicted feelings and values. Imaginal—or Archetypal—psychology is all about this sort of cultivating the rich lived world of a soulful life. Yet in the writings of Hillman and others—especially when read out of context—are echoes of a type of postmodern philosophical groundlessness and solipsism. Unless one acknowledges the gods as beyond one's own soul, then the gods become petty reductions of archetypes, inappropriately constrained to the organs of my psyche. A Jungian might call this being stuck in one's complexes.

The "beyond" to which I appeal here is not just a liberation of the archetypal forces to be more than mere tendencies of my mind. This beyond is that toward which the yearnings of my soul point—toward the edges of what I can know and feel—into Hope and Love and all their glorious and broken manifestations. Spiritual direction invites us to hold our soul's passions up to matters of "Ultimate Concern" as—borrowing from Paul Tillich (1886–1965)—the brilliant and dear John Took says in so many of his existential readings of Dante.

If we can go as deep into our experiences as Zecher's reading of Cassian's vision demands, we may yet reach the level of seeing that to which we have tethered our lives. In doing so, we may release our clutching to smaller things and open up to what cannot be grasped. To my understanding, this is something very much like a transplant; but in this case, it is the removal of a self-inflicted vestigial organ. What remains is an openness to what is beyond our ken. Call it God, or G-d, or the Journey, or the Mystery; but it is what has called us into the room of spiritual direction. It is that into which an empty chair, an opening space, a witnessing director, an icon, a candle, or the ringing of a bell may echo. Perhaps this opening is the Desert into which the Fathers and Mothers as friends to our souls would welcome us.

References

Alighieri, D. (1982). *Inferno* (A. Mandelbaum, Trans.). Bantam Class. (Original work published 1320.)

Barolini, T. (2018). Inferno 13: Non-dualism: our bodies, our selves. *Commento Baroliniano, Digital Dante*. Columbia University Libraries. Available at: https://digitaldante.columbia.edu/dante/divine-comedy/inferno/inferno-13/

Daniels, A. B. (Ed.) (2021). *Dante and the Other: A phenomenology of Love*. Psychology and the Other Series, Routledge.

Hillman, J. (1996). *The soul's code: In search of character and calling*. Random House.

Merton, T. (1960). *The wisdom of the desert: Sayings of the Desert Fathers of the fourth century*. New Directions Books.

O'Donohue, J. (1997). *Anam cara: A book of Celtic wisdom*. Cliff Street Books.

Index

Pages in **bold** refer to tables.

For Product Safety Concerns and Information please contact our EU representative GPSR@taylorandfrancis.com
Taylor & Francis Verlag GmbH, Kaufingerstraße 24, 80331 München, Germany

www.ingramcontent.com/pod-product-compliance
Ingram Content Group UK Ltd.
Pitfield, Milton Keynes, MK11 3LW, UK
UKHW020005200926
475702UK00015B/2481
9781041246336